Food Futures

How Design and Technology can Reshape
our Food System

by Chloé Rutzerveld

B/SPUBLISHERS

BIS Publishers

Building Het Sieraad

Postjesweg 1

1057 DT Amsterdam

The Netherlands

T +31 (0)20 515 02 30

bis@bispublishers.com

www.bispublishers.com

ISBN 978-90-6369-517-0

Copyright © 2018 Chloé Rutzerveld

and BIS Publishers

www.chloerutzerveld.com

Concept, text, design | Chloé Rutzerveld
Art work | Studio Lisa
Editor | Ruben Baart
Proofreading | Jack Caulfield

"Study the science of art. Study the art of science. Develop your senses - especially learn how to see. Realize that everything connects to everything else."

- Leonardo Da Vinci

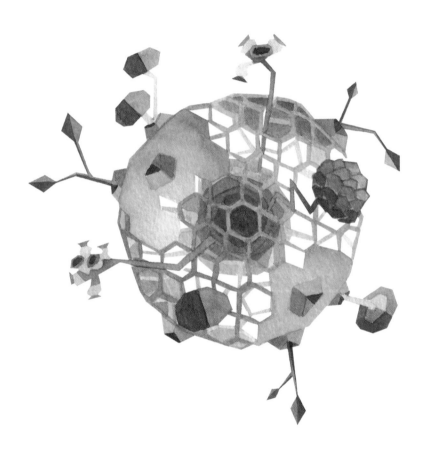

Table of contents

Foreword
Rebecca Chesney

I first came across Chloé's work when she launched Edible Growth in 2014. As a researcher with the Food Futures Lab at the Institute for the Future (IFTF), I was always seeking signals of change—emerging behaviors, technologies, social movements, or business models that pointed to a larger shift in the ways we might produce and consume food. At a time when 3D printing generally recreated familiar foods such as sugar cubes and hamburgers, Chloé was exploring how the technology could enable a new production ecosystem, reimagining the entire process from "planting" seeds to consumption. She demonstrated that new technological capacities open up possibilities for reimagining not just food, but also our relationship with it. When I met Chloé in Bologna, Italy, a few years later, I found a kindred spirit—someone as interested in tradition as innovation, curious what the past can teach us about the future. Chloé's work asks each of us to think beyond what we know today, to imagine what might be tomorrow.

Food Futures chronicles her journey and offers a guide to future food design from the perspective of a visionary practitioner. This book is an important read for anyone interested in food innovation and food systems change.

1. It critically explores alternative futures.

Depending on one's orientation toward technology, science, and food culture, one hears that "the future of food" will be either local, automated, organic, or cultured. Yet such views do not account for the complexity of a global system that already uses a multitude of approaches to produce, manufacture, and cook. With the emergence of indoor farming, synthetic biology, and machine intelligence, our spectrum of options will only become wider. Chloé's projects illuminate the potential edges of that growing spectrum, following the foundations of futures studies laid out by Dr. Jim Dator, Director of the Hawaii Research Center for Futures Studies: (1) that "'the future' cannot be 'predicted,' but 'preferred futures' can and should be envisioned, invented, implemented, continuously evaluated, revised, and re-envisioned," and (2) that "any useful idea about the futures should appear to be ridiculous." As a speculative artist, Chloé's work is provocative, but she makes it a reality today. In this way, she contributes to the community of futurists who illuminate alternative pathways to address the urgent challenges we face now and will continue to face in years to come.

2. It furthers the discipline and practice of food design.
In recent years, a burgeoning community of academics, artists, designers, and culinarians has begun to assert food design as an area for deeper inquiry and exploration. Food design has its own academic conference, peer-reviewed

academic journal (*International Journal of Food Design*), and a magazine that was launched with the help of a Kickstarter crowdfunding campaign (thisismold. com). Inspired by Chloé and her peers, my team with the IFTF Food Futures Lab dedicated a yearlong research project to mapping the intersection of futures thinking and design as a tool to balance opportunities with constraints. Chloé provided her expertise for our research, and with this book, she provides all readers a glimpse of her practice. Through her unique focus on speculative future food design, Chloé shares insight into the challenges of using technologies in ways that are not yet easy to execute. Her solution is to collaborate with plant physiologists, corporate researchers, and DIY biotechnologists, expanding the variety of people who contribute to food design and exemplifying the multidisciplinary, open approaches needed to design a more resilient food system.

3. It invites readers to experience and make the future. As eaters, we influence the future of our food system through the choices we make at each meal. Eating blurs the boundaries between our bodies and the outside world, and forms memories that shape future cravings and behaviors. It's understandably difficult to imagine whether we would eat cultured meat or a dish made from waste if we have never viscerally experienced these foods. In translating her designs into recipes, Chloé invites readers to interact with the future in the present, to deepen their engagement with the unknown and thus deepen the impact of her work. Tapping into food culture, emotions, and aesthetics, Chloé stimulates the changes in mindset that are just as important as changes in technological or scientific capability.

"*Food Futures* is a book for our time and for the years to come. It inspires us to explore the unexpected places innovation will take us if we combine the rigor of scientific inquiry with the reflective nature of art."

Rebecca Chesney
Food Futurist and Innovation Expert

With a background in finance and accounting, international development, and anthropology, Rebecca Chesney maps the forces of change that will impact the global food system. She leads strategic projects with leaders in food R&D, packaging, and marketing to explore possibilities for a more resilient and equitable global food system. Rebecca holds an MA in the Anthropology of Food from SOAS, University of London, and is the former Research Director at the Food Futures Lab at the Institute for the Future.

Introduction

Perhaps you know the feeling. You hear, see or read something, and you cannot let it go. You want to know as much as possible about it, and before you know it, you're connecting everything in your daily surroundings to whatever it is that has caught your attention. Now, your brain is in overdrive and you wake in the middle of the night with a brilliant idea. While you were asleep, your mind processed the information intake from that day and synthesized something new; this new instinct or idea that keeps you up at night, this extreme feeling, paired with a healthy surge of adrenaline, is what drives me as a designer.

Growing up, I was a curious kid with a strong will of my own. I wanted to fiddle all day and enjoyed helping my grandparents in their kitchen garden. But as I grew older, my creativity turned toward science at the urging of my parents. This led me to study Industrial Design at the Eindhoven University of Technology—although honestly, I never really knew what I was doing there. During my studies, I had difficulty persuading myself to learn things that lacked a broad practical application (which, as you may understand, frustrated me a great deal). Everything I created was ugly and did not make any sense to me.

But this all changed in the second year of my studies, when I started a research project focused on growing meat in a laboratory using the stem cells of an animal (as opposed to slaughtering the animal). A method whose product is known as "in vitro meat". The course was led by Dr. Koert van Mensvoort, from Next Nature Network, who challenged his students to dream and speculate about the future, to conceptualize and design scenarios (both utopian and dystopian) that evoked questions, frustrations, fear and fascination in their audiences, and to use "speculative design" as a conversation starter to provoke discussions about the possible futures to which our technological development might lead.

Suddenly I was able to combine my creativity and my interest in nature and food with the world of technology, science and design. It turned out that this entirely new study environment, where experimental research and future thinking were encouraged, was exactly what

I needed to develop myself. Here, I was able to use the freedom of my studies to participate in projects centered on (the future of) food. This resulted in my graduation project Edible Growth, a 3D-printed edible ecosystem. The project received unexpected international acclaim, and launched my career as a food designer.

Food design?

If somebody asks you about your job and you say you work as a firefighter, they will understand what you mean. Answer "food designer", and this understanding is not a given. Food design has become the container concept for all kinds of creative work involving food. Yet there are many different ways to be creative with food; think aesthetics, function, innovation, eating behavior, eating rituals and production processes.

To me, food design means combining science, technology and design to rethink and reflect upon (new) modes of food production and consumption. My projects always take a scientific issue or discovery as their starting point, and aim to bridge the distance between research and production and production and consumption. This way, the consumer is able to experience technological developments in food production in an accessible and interactive way.

To me, food design means combining science, technology and design to rethink and reflect upon modes of food production and consumption.

Food Futures

Welcome to Food Futures, a collection of speculative scenarios that investigate and explore the uncharted possibilities associated with food technologies, and how we can harness these technologies to make our food more healthy, sustainable and efficient. Richly illustrated and vividly narrated from personal experiences, this book contains six chapters—each complemented by stimulating questions, anecdotes and thoughts—designed to work up your appetite. And as I am convinced that "learning by doing" yields better results than passive reading, each chapter contains DIY experiments or recipes which will allow you to experience the food futures at your fingertips.

The structure of this book is as follows. The six chapters are bundled into three parts. The first, Tech for Nature, demonstrates the ways in which the food we eat today is already highly technological. It gives a different perspective on how increasing scientific knowledge—combined with technological development—opens up new ways of producing "natural" food. Tech for Nature shows that design is a powerful tool for involving consumers in scientific research in an accessible way, while at the same time daring scientists and technologists to look ahead.

The second part, Back to the Roots, takes a closer look at what's in our diets, where the ingredients come from, and how we can redefine food waste to increase our health. Moreover, it gives insight into the core question of why we eat in the first place, and how the introduction of a new eating system might affect society as a whole.

By daring to look ahead and envision alternative futures, we can gain new perspective on what we eat, why we do it, and what we may (or may not) eat in the future!

The last part, Beyond Taboos, offers a more forward-facing perspective on how we can overcome cultural taboos to stimulate innovation in science and technology around meat production. It envisions futures involving in vitro meat, explores different ways of introducing the product, and asks the urgent question: If you want to continue eating meat, how far are you prepared to go?

The ultimate goal of this book, then, is to glimpse the possibilities opened up by applying new technologies to our food production, and to show that by daring to look ahead and envision alternative futures, we can gain new perspective on what we eat, why we do it, and what we may (or may not) eat in the future!

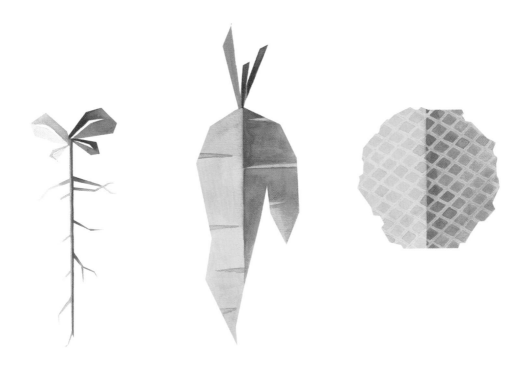

Tech for Nature

1.

Edible Growth

The use of additive manufacturing technologies to create an edible ecosystem.

Agriculture has come a long way since its invention some 10,000 years ago. Industrial farming—once hailed as a technological revolution—is now seen as an outmoded, unsustainable approach to food production. As we humans go about producing and consuming, we set in motion a long list of environmental problems (think air pollution, a plastic soup swirling in the Pacific Ocean, deforestation, animal suffering, climate change). Keeping in mind that the current world population of 7.6 billion is expected to reach 8.6 billion by 2030, 9.8 billion by 2050 and 11.2 billion by 2100, we are in need of new sustainable food production methods that can not only meet global demand, but also minimize our ecological footprint; 3D food printing might be one of the new technologies with the potential to make this possible.

Already in Star Trek: The Next Generation from 1987, we saw crew members of the spaceship "order" their food from the "replicator"; apparently a 3D printer that synthesizes meals on demand. Back then, the idea that a machine could generate a fast, delicious meal from hardly any resources was mind-blowing. But sci-fi narratives like this surely boosted the development of additive manufacturing technologies and might even have inspired scientists to start exploring the printing of food (while the first patent for a 3D printer was filed as early as the 1980s, it took around 30 years for scientists to begin exploring the printing of edible materials). Yet today, it transpires that there is still no "real" food being printed; applications of the technology are limited to decorative cookies, candies and chocolates.

3D-printing food

The first time I encountered printed food was as an attendee of an experimental dinner in 2013. As a dessert, guests were served a 3D-printed chocolate cup filled with vegan ice cream. At that moment, I didn't understand why people were so excited about printed chocolates, cookies and sugar sculptures—and I never have since. They sure look nice, and can be regarded as a first step toward printing a dish that may actually change our eating experience. But at this point, food printers are used mainly as machines for the production of entertaining shapes; ingredient x goes in one side and comes out the other in a different shape. During the process, the quality and flavor of the food can only decrease. I still believe that food printing can radically change the process of getting food from farm to table. But if we're seriously considering food printers as a food production method for the future, we should explore their full potential—as more than just cool gadgets.

Producing healthy food

One year after my encounter with the printed chocolate cup, I was invited by TNO (the Netherlands Organisation for Applied Scientific Research) to think about an innovative 3D-printed food product. As a food printing skeptic, I wasn't sure I was the right person for the job. I didn't want to end up creating yet another ornamental chocolate shape. So I turned the invitation into a challenge: to find a way to use the technology of additive manufacturing—the process of building a three-dimensional object by depositing materials layer by layer—to create healthy food while shortening the food production chain in the process.

As a food printing skeptic, I challenged myself to find a way to use the technology of additive manufacturing to create healthy food while shortening the food production chain in the process.

From limitation to inspiration

A 3D food printer works essentially just like a regular 3D printer. Like its predecessor, the 3D food printer requires materials firm enough to carry themselves, but delicate enough to be pushed through the nozzle.

The most important elements of food printing are:
1. Hardware (the printer)
2. Software (the digital file that tells the printer what to do)
3. A food cartridge (edible printing material)

To print food, you need raw materials. These must be processed into a puree, powder or paste so that the printer can extrude or glue together the food. Especially in case of fruit and vegetables, the processing causes a decrease in nutritional value and a loss of texture. Moreover, it is difficult to print with multiple ingredients at the same time, and because the printer does not bake or cook the food, additional preparation is often still required afterwards.

These limitations explain why it is quite difficult to create healthy food using the techniques currently available. This made my challenge to print healthy food more complicated than I thought it would be. Racking my brain for an ingredient small enough to fit through the printhead so that it wouldn't have to be processed, I suddenly thought: organisms! Because who said the final product had to be fully printed? Why not refigure the printer as a tool to stimulate or even enhance natural growth? What if we printed with organisms such as seeds and spores? These are small enough to pass through the printhead, and could grow into nutritious and crispy food afterwards. A symbiosis between technology and nature. Proof that high-tech food needn't necessarily be artificial and unnatural; instead, technology could support natural growth and bring about exciting, sustainable food innovations.

Imagine a completely edible "mini vegetable garden" with crispy plants and mushrooms; an incomplete dish that becomes a full meal after it has been printed.

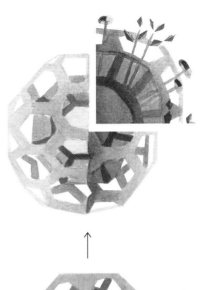

Edible Growth - how it works

Multiple layers containing a basic support structure,
an edible breeding ground and various organisms
are printed directly inside a tiny reusable greenhouse
according to a personalized 3D file. The structure is
designed in such a way that the different organisms
cannot infect each other, but are all able to reach
the breeding ground. After the edible is printed the
consumer places the greenhouse on their windowsill
where sunlight can reach it. The natural process of
photosynthesis begins. Within three to five days, the
plants and mushrooms are fully grown. The intensity
of the taste and smell increases as the dish ripens,
which is also reflected in its changing appearance. The
consumer can decide when to harvest and eat the dish
according to their preferred intensity.

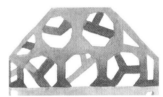

Basic support structure
carbohydrate

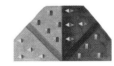

Organisms
spores (Schizophyllum)
seeds (cress)

Edible breeding ground
agar-agar

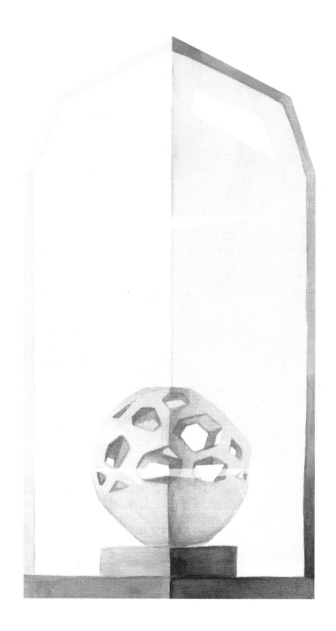

Day one

Print the edible "mini vegetable garden"; an incomplete dish that only becomes a full meal after it has been printed.

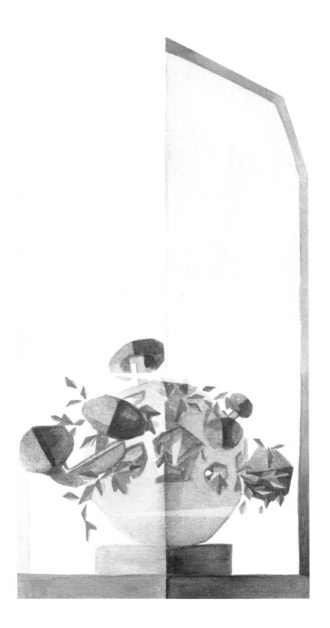

Day five

Nature took over and covered the printed straight lines
with organic growth. It's time to harvest your Edible Growth!

The benefits

Sustainability

• Preventing food waste; because the dish is printed on demand and can only grow after the dry ingredients are mixed with the moisture from the breeding ground.

• No need for packaging as you can reuse the greenhouse.

• Chain shortening; Food grows at home; there is no need for food to travel from the field to the distribution center to the store before finally arriving your home. Reduction of transport emissions as a result.

Consumer involvement

• Closer to the food by seeing the product grow. Experiencing the increase of taste and smell.

• The consumer becomes the farmer and the farmer becomes the supplier of raw materials.

Healthy & fresh

• No cookies, candy or pizza, but healthy food, rich in nutrients with natural textures. Unprocessed, as the dish grows itself.

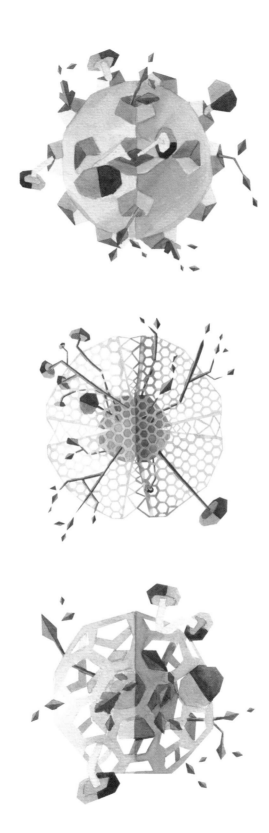

Connecting the dots

For three months I bothered scientists and technologists at TNO with my ambitious plan to print an edible ecosystem. I turned to the microbiologists for knowledge about organisms and edible culture media, and to the technologists for details about printing techniques and their limitations. Combining the insights I sourced from both fields, I came up with new ideas, experiments and questions to develop the concept and aesthetics of Edible Growth further.

After every set of experiments, I went back to the scientists and technologists to ask new questions based on my findings. The design of the edible evolved with each new insight. An external structure with holes at the bottom, for example, is very illogical. Plants and cresses do not grow downward but rather upward, toward the light.

In the beginning of the collaboration, the experts didn't really get it. They often asked, "Why do you want to print an edible ecosystem?" They also found it quite difficult to apply their knowledge to an undertaking with no precedent and for which no preliminary research was available. But in the end, everyone considered the process an inspiring experience and found it refreshing to be taken outside of their daily bubble and look at their profession in a completely novel way.

After a few weeks, I did have to face the facts and realize that the concept of Edible Growth was a little more complex than I had initially assumed—partly due to my own limited knowledge of microbiology, but also due to the limitations of the printing technology. Fortunately, it was never my goal to bring a 3D-printed product to the market; the goal was to envision an alternative way of using printing techniques to produce healthy food and shorten the production chain.

The design evolved with each new insight.

An external structure with holes at the bottom, for example, is very illogical.

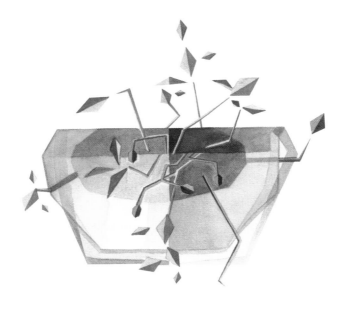

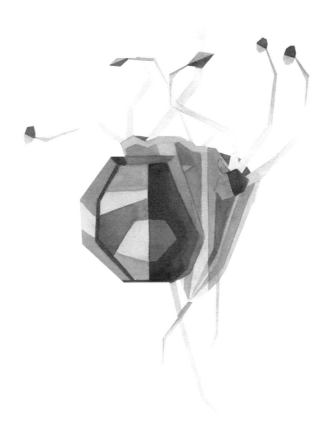

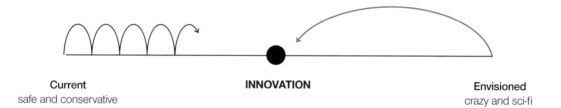

Current
safe and conservative

INNOVATION

Envisioned
crazy and sci-fi

A speculative road to innovation

I always start my design process from the envisioned side—to prevent
practical complications in the 'here and now' from imagining 'what could be'
in the future. Once I have found my solution or idea, I go back one step to
think about what needs to be done in order to make it happen.

The power of speculative design and strong images

As I was unable to print and grow a real Edible Growth, I decided to make the most realistic prototypes I could. Using a powder-bed printed outer frame wrapped in dough, then baked in the oven, I filled the cups with Enoki and Shimeji mushrooms and tufts of garden cress. By varying the size and quantity of the mushrooms, I could simulate the growth process of Edible Growth in steps and create a stop-motion video of the growth.

The level of photorealism in the pictures and video was rather high, and it was immediately assumed that Edible Growth was possible, resulting in a viral project circulating on the internet and becoming one of the top hits on Google when searching for "3D printing" and "food"—ironic, as I was still skeptical about printing food and had never touched a 3D printer myself.

From this project, I learned the importance of good images and the need for creativity and innovative thinking in the food industry. What I had also gained was an understanding of how to make an impact with little to no funding but limitless curiosity, creativity and perseverance. Apparently bread dough, mushrooms, and a good photo can get you pretty far.

You don't need a lot of money to make an impact on the world

What you need is curiosity, creativity and perseverance.
(and a bit of bread dough)

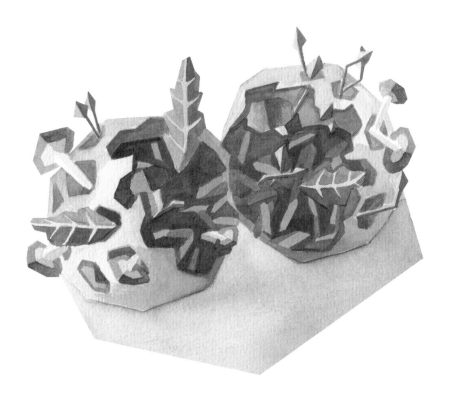

A conceptual eating experience

Edible Growth-inspired mushroom risotto with red wine

Food is a very powerful means of communication. What we have seen so far is that, while
the real product cannot be made yet due to its speculative nature, it's the story, and giving the
audience an idea of how the product might look and taste in the future, that counts. I often
serve Edible Growth as a main course during an experimental dinner. To make it a filling meal,
I supplement the plants and mushrooms with a forest mushroom risotto cooked in red wine,
topped off with cress and arugula. By serving the whole under a dome, I allow condensation to
form on the glass, making it seem like a real greenhouse in which the Edible Growth has grown.

Instructions

Prepare four portions of red wine mushroom risotto. Take the dough out of the freezer and separate the sheets to defrost. Preheat the oven to 180 °C.

1. Top part of the Edible Growth (x4) | Use the glass to cut a circle in the dough and use the diamond-shaped cutter to cut out the holes for the dome. Place the incised dough circle over the curved side of the mold. Repeat three times. When finished, put the mold into the oven and bake for 15 minutes until the domes are baked and slightly tanned. Take the mold out of the oven and let it cool before taking off the dough.

2. Base part of the Edible Growth (x4) | Fold a sheet of dough over the curved side of the mold. Use a knife to cut off the additional dough to create a nice cup. Repeat three times. Bake for 15 minutes at 180 °C. Again, let the mold cool before taking off the dough.

3. Mise en place | Cut and clean as many mushrooms as you like to decorate four Edible Growth baskets. Mix the olive oil, apple cider vinegar, lemon juice, salt and pepper in a bowl to create the marinade. Carefully add the mushrooms and let them marinade for at least 10 minutes.

4. Finish the dish | Place the base cup on the bottom part of the glass bell and fill it with mushroom risotto. Take the top part of the crust and place it on the base part to form a ball. Stick some Enoki and Shimeji mushrooms inside the holes and add a few arugula leaves and puffs of cress to finish the dish. Cover it with the glass bell. Your Edible Growth is ready to be served!

Ingredients (4 pers.)

- 8 sheets frozen savory pie dough
- 1 bag of small arugula leaves
- 1 box of Shimeji mushrooms
- 1 box of Enoki mushrooms
- 1 box of cress
- pinch salt and pepper
- 1 tbs olive oil
- 1 tsp lemon juice
- 2 tbs apple cider vinegar
- 4 portions of red wine mushrooom risotto

Material

- silicone half sphere molds (ø 7cm)
- diamond-shaped cutter (ø 1cm)
- glass (top part ø 9cm)
- knife
- tweezers
- bowl for marinade
- spoon
- 4x glass bell for serving

2.
Future Food Formula
Design your own vegetable with the use of growth recipes.

Traditional farming is highly climate-dependent. A sudden cold snap can seriously damage crops in a short period of time. The possibility of growing crops indoors, unaffected by weather conditions, means not having to depend on specific regions of the globe to supply the majority of our produce. Decentralizing food production makes sense in terms of feeding a growing population, but can also reduce food miles (the distance food travels from where it's grown to where it's consumed) and the carbon footprint. Plus, the fresher the produce, the more nutrients it holds and the better it tastes.

Perhaps you've heard of vertical farming, a technology that allows stacks of plants to grow in an indoor environment. Initially, I never had much interest in indoor growing systems. Only after I got the chance to taste the perfect lettuce did I become curious about the possibilities of this technology. I was intrigued to learn about the important role that the application of different LED colors plays in the development of the crops. But what fascinated me most was the notion of a "growth recipe."

Simulating the perfect growth environment

It may seem logical to us that a tomato grown in Spain is redder, juicier, and richer in taste than it would be were it grown in the Netherlands; Spain has a warmer climate, and the crops get more hours of sunlight. But these are just a few of the factors that influence the growing process. As I dove into vertical farming technology, I discovered that it is not only the amount of sun and water that impacts the development of a crop; factors such as humidity, airflow, light spectrum, CO_2 concentration and the pH value of the soil are equally important. In fact, the adjustment of one growing factor can influence the shape, size, color, smell, taste, texture and nutritional value of a crop.

Inside high-tech growth facilities, each of these environmental factors can be simulated and determined separately. The values are written down in so-called "growth recipes." Because tomato plants react differently to certain environmental factors than lettuce, scientists create a specific recipe for each crop. This way, the farmer can decide either to grow the crop in its regular growth cycle, or to optimize the growing conditions in order to increase the quality of the crop or incite higher yields.

Growth recipes, revisited

In summary, vertical farming technology enables us to grow perfect crops; it helps us make optimal use of resources and reduces agricultural land use, while enabling the production of local and fresh food. Cultivating perfect crops will surely prevent a lot of food waste, but mightn't this uniformity become boring in the long run? What if we explored the limits of this technology and experimented with the use of growth recipes for purposes other than efficiency?

Already when adapting a recipe to our own liking, we adjust the taste, smell, color and nutritional value of the dish. But what if technology could allow us to do the same thing directly to our crops? This would mean that in the future, we could "cook" with growth recipes instead of with ingredients. We simply compile a growth recipe that contains our preferences before the seed even grows; this will bring forth a new generation of crops through experimental growth recipes.

How can we create new generations of crops through experimental growth recipes?

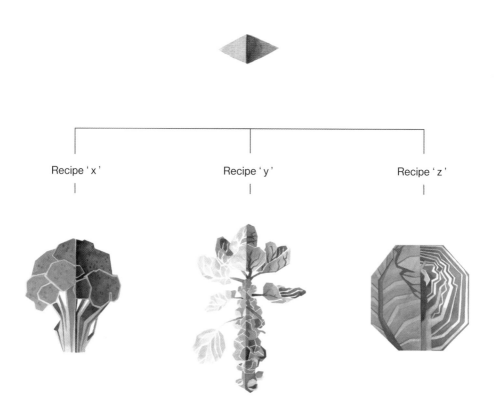

Recipe 'x'   Recipe 'y'   Recipe 'z'

Scenario one - Whimsical seed

All cabbages—think cauliflower, Brussels sprouts, kale and broccoli—
are "spontaneous" mutations originating from the same cabbage-like
ancestor. What if one seed held all the genetic information to grow all
family members, depending on what growth recipe you apply?

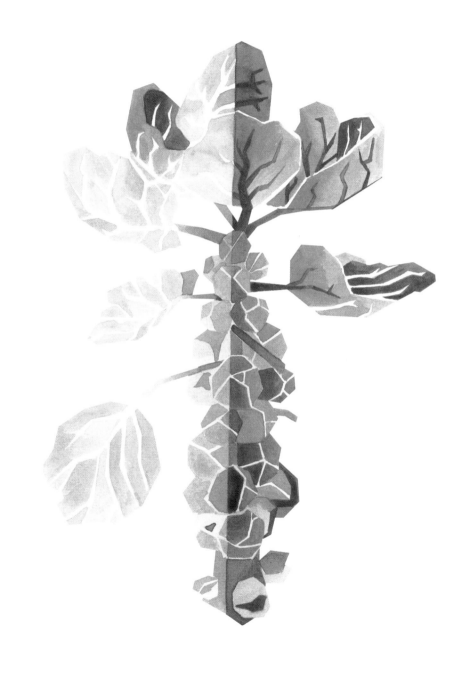

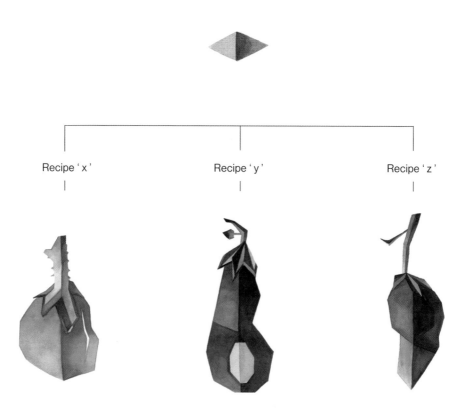

Recipe ' x '   Recipe ' y '   Recipe ' z '

Scenario two - Infinity seed

Grow unlimited variations of one specific crop by experimenting
with the variables in the recipe. Design crops with new flavors,
shapes, textures and colors, and share your creations with the world.

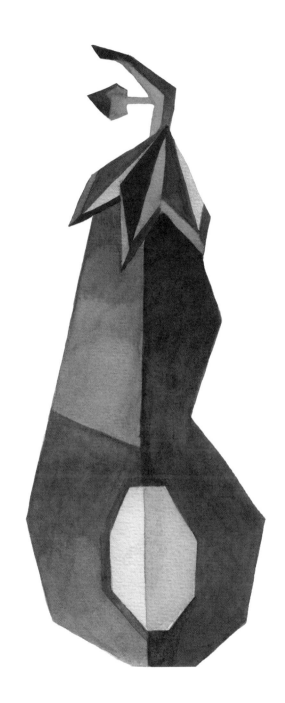

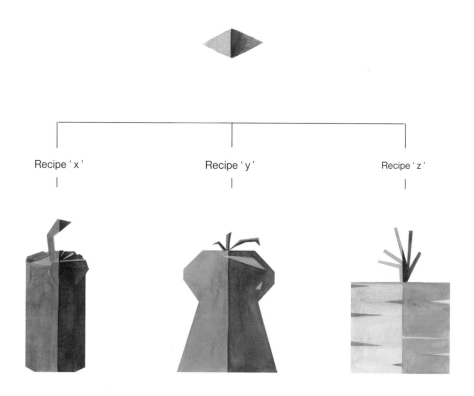

Recipe ' x '

Recipe ' y '

Recipe ' z '

Scenario three - Geometry seed

Grow functional vegetables to reduce food waste and increase
efficiency. Meet the "sandwich tomatoes" and "cylindrical eggplants."

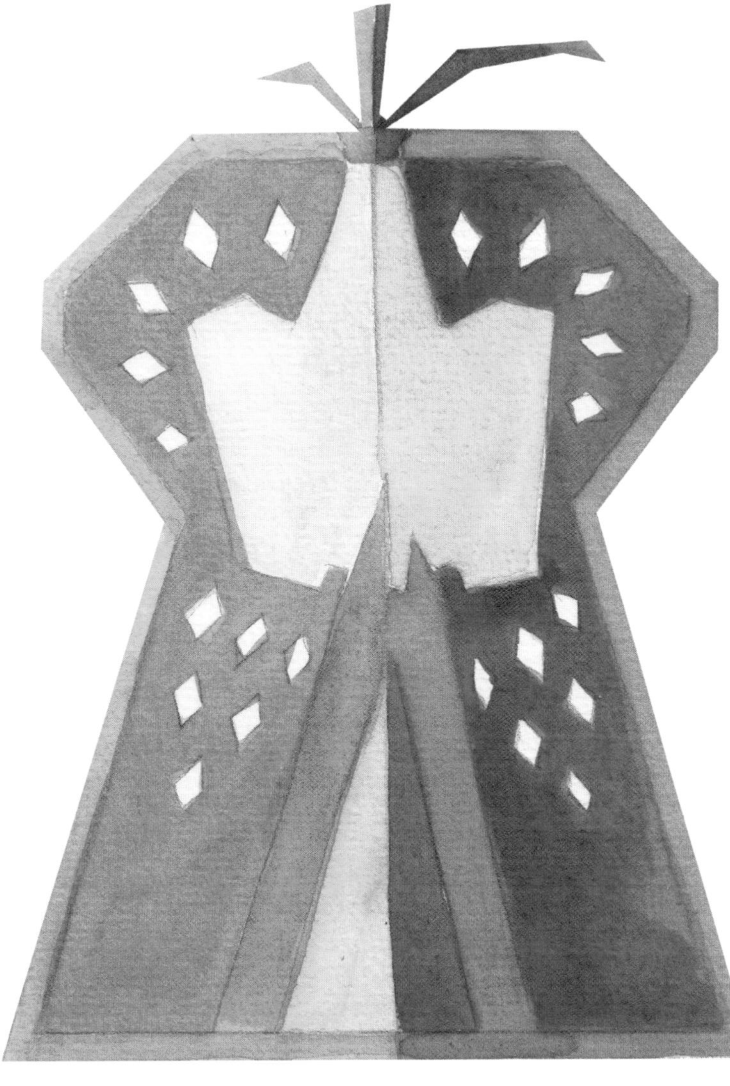

All our food is highly technological. So why do we still hold on to this romantic idea of the farmer in the small field?

Altering phenotypes

If all our food is already highly technological, why hold on to this romantic idea of the farmer in the small field? Instead, let's use all the knowledge and expertise out there to produce next-level crops that reduce labor intensity, food waste and costs. In doing so, one could imagine a slice of "sandwich tomato," or a julienne "carrot cube" that saves chefs hours of carving time. Or what about "doubter seeds" that grow into either broccoli, cauliflower or Brussels sprouts, depending on the growth recipe the consumer applies?

Admittedly, many of these scenarios are still highly speculative, and they can't be achieved on short notice without the use of genetic modification. But we can already begin to look forward, exploring how we can change our crops without genetic modification, purely by experimenting with growth recipes. So I started researching the influence of different growth factors on the phenotypes (the observable characteristics of an individual crop resulting from its interaction with the environment) of crops.

As many factors play a role, I decided to focus on the following six factors:

- light spectrum (red, far red, blue, UV light)
- light intensity
- pH
- CO_2
- air temperature
- water

Since I am not a (plant) biologist myself, I collaborated with the Association for Vertical Farming, a master's student in plant physiology at Wageningen University, and a researcher from Philips Lighting. Looking at each factor in turn, we asked ourselves what functionality it had, how it would affect crops at both high and low intensity, and how this would influence the nutritional value of the plant. Having obtained all of this crop data, I created an overview that gives insight into how each growth factor influences the crops. This data became the starting point for the development of an interactive installation: The Future Food Formula.

The influence of growth factors on crop development

This overview gives a general idea of how plant physiology and the natural manipulation of crops works. An increase or decrease in one parameter can directly necessitate a change in another parameter to prevent the crop from dying. For example, when you increase the amount of red light—which activates plant growth—you will also need to increase the concentration of CO_2 to enable higher photosynthesis levels, and increase the amount of water to prevent the crop from drying out.

	Red light	Far-red light	Blue light
Function	Red light promotes plant growth (stem, leaves, fruits) by activating the production of chloroplasts. Chloroplasts are needed to absorb light and convert it into the chemical energy needed for photosynthesis. Through the photosynthesis process, the sugars which allow the plant to grow are produced.	In nature, when plants are shaded by neighboring plants, they receive a lot of far-red light. If the ratio between red and far-red light is out of proportion (far-red > red) then the shade-avoidance syndrome appears. To compete for light, the plants use all their energy for elongation. The physical stress also stimulates the production of antioxidants and volatile compounds—which increases the taste, nutritional value and aroma of the plant.	Like red light, blue light is responsible for photosynthesis and the production of chlorophyll in the leaves. For efficient photosynthesis, a good ratio between blue and red light is desirable (red > blue). Blue light boosts the absorption and production of micro-nutrients.
High intensity	High photosynthesis rate, so faster development and growth of the crop. Required: increased level of CO_2 and water. High intensity of red light also promotes the development of branches. The produced crop will be much bigger, sweeter and with an airier texture.	Elongation of the plant. Stems: long, thin. Leaves: larger surface to catch more light; leaves tilt upwards; thinner; lighter color due to inactive phytochrome which reduces the chlorophyll. Crop: longer and smaller than with a normal ratio or red light, but tastier.	When blue light > red light, blue light has a negative effect on photosynthesis. Stems, leaves and fruits become smaller, firmer and denser. However, as a result the amount of nutrients, antioxidants and flavor all increase. Plants grow toward blue light, so when blue light comes from the side it causes crooked growth and distortion.
Low intensity	Little to no red light slows down the photosynthesis process and therefore crop growth. If the development of the chloroplasts is also disrupted, mutations appear in the leaves and they develop white or yellow spots due to a lack of chlorophyll production. The produced crop will be smaller, and less sweet	The stems, leaves and fruits are thicker and more compact. Leaves are much darker because there is more chlorophyll present. Absence of red light slows down crop growth and reduces nutritional value.	Little or no blue light reduces the absorption and production of antioxidants and polyphenols (substances in the peel of the fruit or vegetable which influence taste and enable mineral absorption).

Stressed plants taste better.

Did you know you can increase the flavor and aromatic levels of herbs such as basil and oregano by creating 'stressful' growing conditions? High light intensity, dryness, warm temperatures and high rates of airflow will concentrate the essential oils in the leaves. Because volatile compounds are related to flavor; the higher the concentration of essential oils, the richer the flavor of the herbs!

	UV light	Light intensity	CO_2
Function	Similar to how it affects our own skin, UV light affects the pigments of the crop and influences the color of the fruit, flower, leaves and stems. It can cause DNA damage and morphing, a decrease in flowering and pollination, and can also reduce the photosynthesis rate, affecting the plant mass. Exposure to visible violet light, however, may enhance taste, aroma, and color.	In general, the more light a plant receives, the faster it grows—although this strongly depends on the ratio of the different light spectrums, the amount of CO_2 and water and the temperature. High amounts of light but a low CO_2 concentration, not enough water and temperatures too cold or too hot can cause growth to stagnate or even kill the plant. (standard = 200 umol/m2/s)	Plants need CO_2 for the photosynthesis process to produce energy (glucose) to grow: water + CO_2 + light = glucose and oxygen. The concentration of CO_2 therefore influences the efficiency and speed of photosynthesis and thus how fast the plant grows. However, if other conditions are unfavorable, the effect is negligible. (standard = 400ppm)
High intensity	The color intensifies and becomes darker. Reduction of photosynthesis rate affects the plant mass. High quantities of UV light cause mutations and morphing of crops. Extremely high quantities cause scorch marks or even burn the plants entirely.	High intensity 600 - 1000 umol/m2/s causes a decrease in quality of the fruit: cracking, burn spots, uneven ripeness. As light stimulates the production of chlorophyll (responsible for the green color of the leaves) leaves becomes darker. Additionally, the quantity of leaves increases, as there is more light to catch.	When CO_2 concentration > 400 ppm, it can speed up photosynthesis, promoting plant growth and branching.
Low intensity	Just a little bit of UV light during a short period of time results in healthier fruits, with beautifully bright colors. It enriches the production of antioxidants and the absorption of minerals.	Low light intensity <50 umol/m2/s causes small crops because of slow photosynthetic rate. There is little production of leaves and chlorophyll, because there is no light to catch. Leaves that are present will grow a bigger surface instead. There is a possibility that crops don't grow, or don't flower at all.	When the CO_2 concentration drops below 400 ppm, it slows down photosynthesis and plant growth.

pH	Air temperature	Water
The pH (often determined by the electrolytes inside the water) influences the absorption of nutrients by the plant. An ideal pH is between 5.5 and 6.2. *(standard 5.5)*	Temperature regulates the biorhythm of the crop. It is important that the temperature during the night is lower than during the day, so that the plant can cool off. This is important for the development of the fruit and the overall growth of the plant. *(standard for tomato-like plant 25 °C)*	The amount of water influences the growth of the crop, its shape and nutritional value. The perfect amount of water varies for every crop and is highly dependent on other growth conditions.
When the pH is very basic (> 6.5), it is difficult for the roots of the plant to absorb micronutrients such as copper, iron, magnesium and zinc. This can cause a nutrient deficiency in the plant. The leaves become yellow or white.	Temperatures of 30 °C and up negatively influence flowering and crop development. Temperatures above 35 °C cause paleness, discoloration and water stress. The fruits and leaves lose their firmness and become brown and soft. Eventually dehydration, abnormal seed formation and blossom end rot occur.	A lot of water, but not too much will slow down the development of the crop. Too much water causes a shortage of oxygen which means that the roots will die. Overwatering increases mold growth and other diseases can make the crop crack.
When the pH is very acidic (< 5.0), crops can become sour or even toxic. Fruits and leaves show symptoms of deteriorating calcium and magnesium intake (ugly spots on leaves and on the crop, color changes).	Temperatures below 14 °C slow down the growth process. Below 10 °C, plants stop growing and become non-active until conditions improve.	When the plant doesn't receive enough water, stress will occur. The plant will have a decreased ability to absorb nutrients because of dehydration. The crop can also rot, or simply die.

Function

High intensity

Low intensity

We will start cooking with growth recipes instead of with ingredients.

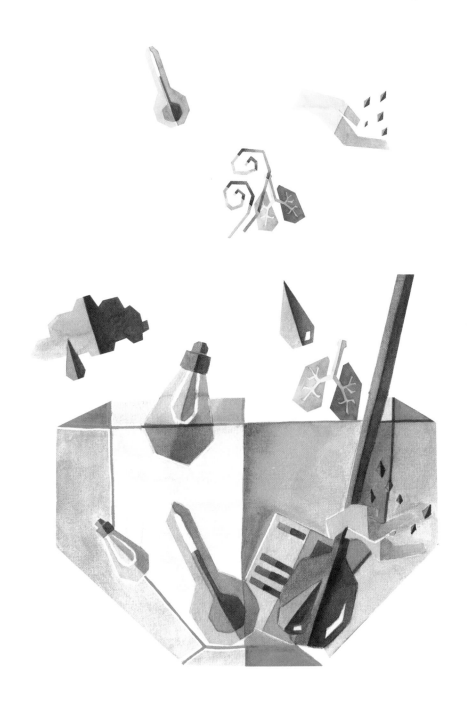

Cooking with growth recipes

Future Food Formula

All too often, consumers learn about a new technology only when the product is already on the market. Because research on novelty foods and new technology is not openly accessible or is too complex for regular consumers to understand, there is often a lack of communication. This problem demonstrates the enormous gap between research, development and consumption; if the consumers are the ones who buy and consume the food, wouldn't it make sense to involve them at an earlier stage?

I felt therefore that it was time to translate this knowledge into an approachable, interactive installation, enabling the consumer to learn about indoor farming technology and plant physiology while playfully designing their own future crop. As consumers adjust the amount of CO2, temperature and light on a touchscreen interface, they see how their adaptations impact the shape, size and color of the crop.

Design your own vegetable by adjusting the growth recipe.

To realize the Future Food Formula, the textual research had to be translated into visual data. To begin, I designed a basic model with standard growing conditions (Recipe 001) that resembled a fictitious crop. For every factor (light, pH, temperature, etc.) I made two 2D drawings that visualized how each parameter would influence the crop at minimum and maximum intensity.

After having transformed all data into 2D drawings, I collaborated with a modelling artist to create 3D sketches. Studio RNDR processed these sketches into a computer-generated responsive model. This model merges the forms and morphs them into new crops, depending on the values entered into the growth recipe on the interface. To enrich the consumer experience, the Future Food Formula showcases eight possible outcomes for futuristic crops; same seeds, different vegetables.

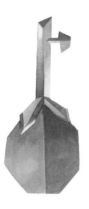

Recipe 001

Red light 60%

Far-red light 15%

Blue light 30%

UV light 0%

Temperature 25°C

CO_2 400ppm

pH 5.5

Water 110ml

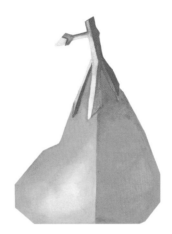

Recipe 087

Red light 98%

Far-red light 10%

Blue light 30%

UV light 0%

Temperature 28°C

CO_2 622ppm

pH 5.5

Water 246ml

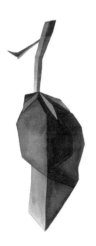

Recipe 042

Red light 42%

Far-red light 15%

Blue light 36%

UV light 95%

Temperature 23°C

CO_2 484ppm

pH 5.5

Water 70ml

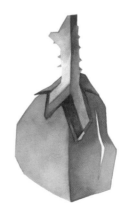

Recipe 038

Red light 60%

Far-red light 10%

Blue light 30%

UV light 0%

Temperature 25°C

CO_2 676ppm

pH 5.5

Water 230ml

Decentralized plant breeding

Now it's up to the scientists to experiment with the growth recipes and see whether it's possible to grow different phenotypes, flavors and nutritional values from just one seed, based on the applied growing conditions. If this works, we can all welcome a climate-controlled cultivation system into our kitchen and start experimenting for ourselves.

This may lead to a future of decentralized plant breeding. We may be able to design and grow new generations of crops from our homes, and upload (or download) the growth recipes onto a digital server, from which—based on the amount of "likes" or "shares" each recipe receives—producers can pick out which crops they want to mass-produce.

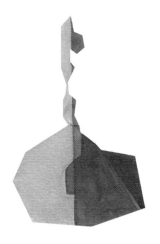

 30   58

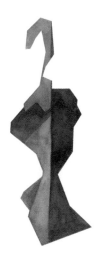

 18   24

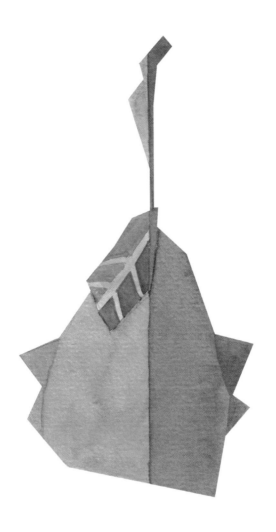

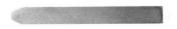

DOWNLOADING 63%

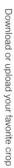

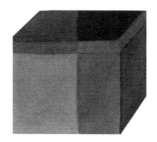

Recipe 042

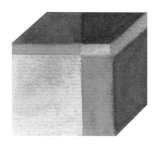

Recipe 001

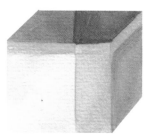

Recipe 087

A taste of the future
Create and compare future crops

As computer visualizations happen on screens, they're not ideal for communicating smell, taste, texture and nutritional value. That's why I've developed three recipes to give you a taste of the future crops: a combination of familiar current-day vegetables to simulate the creation of new vegetables. For the best experience, make all three crops and organize a tasting session—this way you can taste, smell, feel and see the difference between the crops!

Red is the basic crop, while orange is a very thick, large, sweet and airy crop that has received a lot of CO_2, red light and water. Purple is a mashed crop with crazy shapes, small, compact, high in nutritional value because it has received a lot of blue light and UV light during the growth process.

Instructions

Note: The instructions and tools for making the purple and orange crop are exactly the same, only with different ingredients. These are listed on the next page.

Preheat the oven to 200 °C. Cut the eggplant, bell pepper and tomatoes in half and put them in an oven dish. Leave the vegetables in the oven for 30 minutes until softened.

1. Making the crop | Place the eggplant, tomato and 100 grams of the bell pepper in a bowl. Puree the vegetables with a blender, add the flour and baking powder to the bowl, while using a spoon or whisk to mix everything together. Beat the eggs in a different bowl before adding them to the mixture. Cover the mold with baking paper and pour the vegetable mix into the mold. Put the mold in the preheated oven and bake the "crop" at 200 °C for 30 minutes.

2. Making the 'peel' of the crop | Start making the peel once the crop part is finished and has cooled off. Blend the remaining 75 grams of bell pepper with the blender in a small pan. Add 1/3 cup of water and 2 tsp agar. Bring the mixture to a boil while stirring. Continue boiling and stirring for two more minutes. Switch off the heat and let the "peel mixture" cool while you keep stirring. Wait before applying the peel layer to the crop part until the liquid begins to solidify. Now pour the liquid on top of the crop part and use the back side of a spoon to even the layer. Carefully place the mold inside the refrigerator for at least 30 minutes to let the agar peel set. When all three future crops are done, take them out of the refrigerator and cut them into small square pieces for the tasting session.

Ingredients

(+/- 20 blocks)

Red "crop"

- 135 g eggplant
- 175 g red bell pepper
- 100 g tomato
- 50 g spelt flour
- 50 g self-rising wheat flour
- 2 eggs
- 2 tsp agar powder
- 1/3 cup of water

Material

- cake mold 30cm x 20cm
- baking paper
- blender
- big bowl
- oven dish
- saucepan
- scale
- spoon
- whisk

Purple "crop"

Ingredients crop

- 300 g eggplant, softened in oven
- 50 g self-rising wheat flour
- 50 g spelt flour
- 2 eggs, beaten
- ½ tbs blackberry marmelade
- ½ tbs cacao powder

Ingredients peel

- 30 g eggplant, softened in oven
- 1/3 cup of water
- ½ tbs blackberry marmelade
- 2 tsp agar powder

Orange "crop"

Ingredients crop

- 50 g bell pepper, softened in oven
- 200 g pumpkin, softened in oven
- 50 g strawberries (fresh or frozen)
- 100 g self-rising wheat flour
- 2 eggs, beaten
- ½ tsp baking powder

Ingredients peel

- 70 g pumpkin, softened in oven
- 1/3 cup of water
- 2 tsp agar powder

The orange crop, sliced open

Back to
the Roots

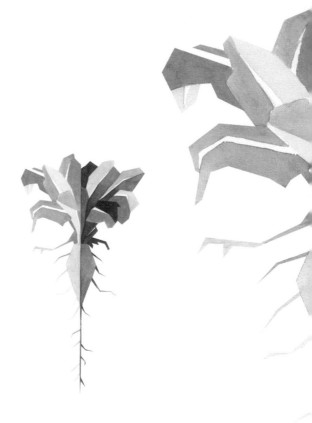

3.

STROOOP!

How does our perception of an ingredient change from "healthy and natural" to "unhealthy and unnatural"?

For many products we simply know whether it's healthy or unhealthy; a carrot is clearly healthy, and a sweet fizzy drink is not, right? We grow up learning that fruit and vegetables are good for us, and that pastries, sweets and chips are not and should be consumed with moderation. As it turns out, it's not as simple as that.

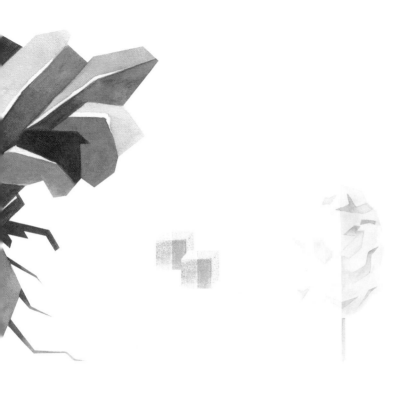

Some time ago, when I was preparing sweet potatoes in the oven, I noticed a thick caramel-like substance running out of them. It was an incredibly sweet syrup, which made me reconsider my view on sweet potatoes as "healthy"; how could something as sweet as candy still be considered a healthy vegetable? Knowing that tuberous plants such as (sweet) potatoes, beets and carrots contain lots of carbohydrates, I realized that these carbohydrates are in fact built from sugars, starches and fibers. Heating the potatoes caused the complex carbohydrate chains (disaccharides) to break down into simpler glucose molecules (monosaccharides, 2x glucose), which resulted in the sweet potato releasing its sugars and "becoming sweet" during the baking process. I wondered why

I had never asked myself what exactly was inside the raw ingredients I'm eating, and realized that each processing method has a different effect on the nutritional value of the food.

Struck by my own astonishment and the extreme sweetness of the potato, I got thinking about how consumer perception of a given product could shift from "healthy and natural" to "unhealthy and unnatural." If we were to take the natural sweetness of the potato, and turn it into a completely different "type" of product, with virtually no additives, would people then—regardless of the type of product—consider it healthy, because it's entirely made from vegetables?

A cotton candy fantasy

Cotton candy is undoubtedly the opposite of a healthy product. So how better to question the large amount of sugar present inside the sweet potato than by turning it into cotton candy? And so, the challenge and experimentation began.

Yet as cotton candy is made from sucrose (the sugar crystals you put into your coffee), and the sugar present in sweet potatoes is maltose (which is glucose), the experiment didn't succeed. It was technically impossible to make cotton candy out of a sweet potato, as you cannot make sugar crystals from glucose. On the advice of a plant biologist I turned to carrots and beets, as these do contain sucrose. But these experiments also failed due both to applying the wrong method and to a lack of equipment— and patience. However, what I learned from these failed experiments was how to generate delicious vegetable syrups, with a stack of fibers as a residual product.

Considering my initial challenge was to use a single portion of a root vegetable to create an entirely different product, the fibers also had to be processed into the final product. Suddenly it became clear: Why not make vegetable stroopwafels? A modern, plant-based version of a typical Dutch delicacy (two waffles with a layer of syrup in between). A radiant way to communicate the story; stroopwafels are familiar, loved by many, and most importantly, delicious!

How can we turn one portion of root vegetable into one stroopwafel by making smart use of its natural properties?

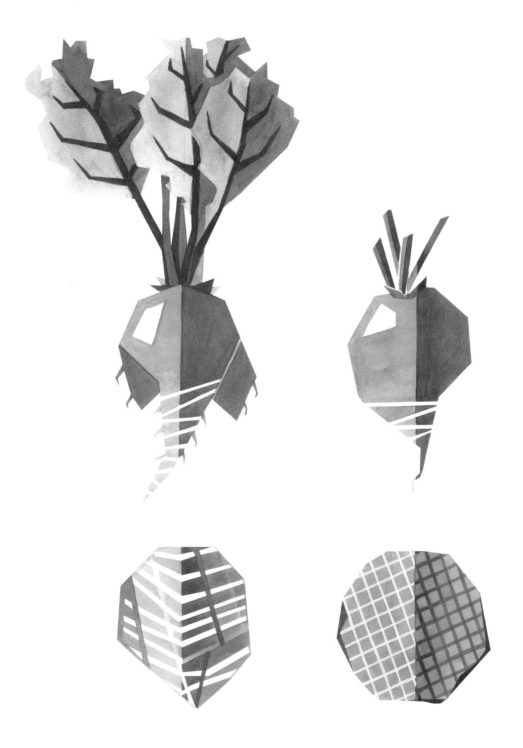

55

From waste to waffle

Making vegetable syrup was the easy part; you simply reduce the water content of the juice until you're left with a high viscosity sugar substance. Creating a crispy waffle from a pile of fibers was not so simple. The ratio between the juice (for the syrup) and fiber (for the dough) had to be just right to make it work. Therefore, I had to test a whole range of root vegetables to determine which would create the tastiest syrup and give the best yield. For example, onion leaves virtually no fibers, it's mainly juice and has a very intense aroma and flavor. Celeriac, on the other hand, contains little juice, leaves a very sturdy syrup, and contains a lot of fiber. During the testing period, I experimented with onion, Jerusalem artichoke, potato, sweet potato, celeriac, beet, carrot, parsnip, but also other crops such as pumpkin and bell pepper. In the end I chose to continue with carrots and beetroots; these had the best combination of taste, color, ratio and yield.

Once I had found the right method and ingredients, I gained a new perspective. I figured, if I needed the fibers and juice separate anyway, why not work with waste products? Just think of the amount of rejected vegetables that simply don't make it to the supermarkets because they don't meet the "standard," or the large quantities of residual flows wasted during the processing of pre-packaged vegetable wedges? This project was the perfect occasion to experiment with waste streams, turning them into interesting consumer products by making smart use of their natural properties.

I figured, if I needed the fibers and juice separate anyway, why not work with waste products?

So I collaborated with Proverka, an agricultural company that grows and processes vegetables, but also creates vegetable juices and fibers from residual flows. During the project, they supplied the fiber and the juice from beets and carrots. As mentioned, it was quite the challenge to turn a pile of fiber into a nice waffle that can be sliced like a "normal" stroopwafel. To improve the crispiness and functionality of the waffle, I worked with a master's student in Food Technology at Wageningen University. Crispiness and fiber don't really match well; fibers attract moisture from their surroundings, causing the waffle to lose its crunch within fifteen minutes.

We therefore needed to create a barrier, either by adding sugar to the dough, coating the waffle, or with airtight packaging. However, none of these options suited the goal of the project—which was, after all not to create a vegetable stroopwafel from waste, but to explore what else can be made from beetroot or carrot (it could easily have been any other product). To continue with the stroopwafel as our means of communication, we agreed to serve it exclusively as a fresh product, to be eaten directly after production.

Syrup

About 78% exists out of
juice, from which 6 grams of
vegetable syrup can be made.
Without added sugar of course.

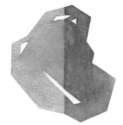

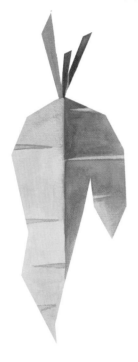

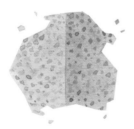

Stroopwafel 1:1

After the waffle is baked, it's
sliced open and covered with a
layer of vegetable syrup.
Et voilà; one stroopwafel made
from vegetable by-products.

Vegetable

100 grams of weird, damaged
or leftover vegetables are
cleaned and juiced.

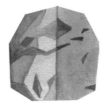

Dough

The remaining 22% consists of
fiber. To transform the fiber into
dough for the waffle, a little bit
of buckwheat flour, rapeseed
oil and salt is added.

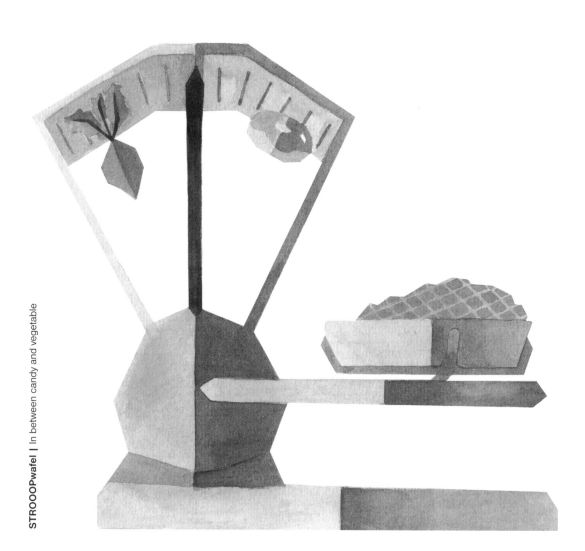

STROOOP! - The project

The project explores creative ways to turn byproducts of the vegetable industry into high-quality products by making smart use of the natural characteristics of vegetables. It demonstrates that the use of byproducts and rejected vegetables can go far beyond making boring soups and sauces. At the same time, it educates the consumer about what's inside our food and questions their perception of certain products.

STROOOP! presents the first plant-based stroopwafel made from local byproducts of the Dutch vegetable industry. Each waffle is made out of 100 grams of carrot or beetroot. They are a great source of dietary fiber and free of gluten, added sugar and food-colorings.

The impact on the consumer

My starting question—candy or vegetable?—was a hard one to answer. Because we had to add some flour and oil, technically it was no longer entirely made from vegetable matter. The public therefore saw it as a healthier and more sustainable version of the stroopwafel; a product somewhere in between a vegetable and a fatty, sugary snack.

Many parents were surprised to see their kids—who normally don't want to eat carrots or beets—enjoyed the vegetable stroopwafels. Moreover, they found it difficult to believe that the sweet syrup was made purely from reduced beet or carrot juice. The waffles proved to be an accessible way for kids to learn to eat vegetables and increase their fiber consumption. Because with 100 grams of vegetable matter in every waffle, you can still taste the carrot or beetroot—but of course in a less intense way than when eating the raw vegetable.

The public saw the STROOOP-wafel as a product somewhere in between a vegetable and a fatty, sugary snack.

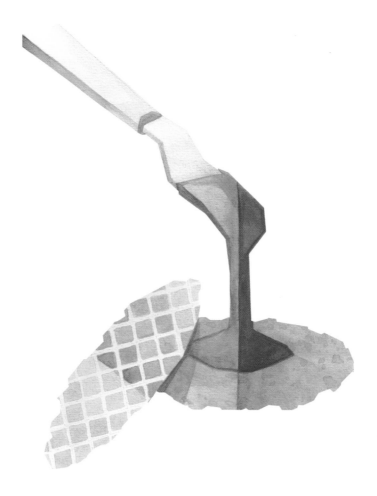

Recipe | Vegetable stroopwafel

Not every carrot or beet has the same water content. The recipe for the waffle therefore cannot be standardized when using the fiber and juice from whole produce. It might take some trial and error before you end up baking the perfect waffle. But, that's great; this recipe is only supposed to help you with your experimentation anyway. If you only mix and bake one waffle at a time, it's easy to adjust the recipe for the next waffle if the mixture was too sticky, wet or dry.

Mix it up! Once you feel comfortable experimenting with the basic waffles, you can basically create any kind of stroopwafel you can think of! What about a fresh summer variation with cucumber, fennel, mint and pineapple syrup? Or turning your favorite dish into a stroopwafel? Just imagine what a spaghetti Bolognese stroopwafel would taste like...

Instructions

Note: the same method applies for beetroots and celeriac.

Wash the carrots and cut them into pieces that fit into your juicer. Separate the juice from the fiber. After juicing, put the fiber into the nut milk bag or a clean dish towel and squeeze out as much of the leftover juice (into the juice bowl) as you can. You want the fiber to be as dry as possible; the drier the fiber, the crunchier your waffle will be.

Making the syrup | Filter the juice by pouring it through the sieve inside the pan. Bring the juice to a boil while whisking. Continue whisking on high heat to evaporate the water from the juice. Tip: this might go faster if you switch your extractor fan to the highest level. You will notice some foam floating on top of the liquid; this is a mixture of denatured proteins and carotene. Carotene is responsible for the orange color of carrots and many other fruits, vegetables and even some animals. Use the sieve to remove the foam from the pan, to keep your syrup clear. When you have evaporated around 90% of the liquid the syrup will be almost done. First, the consistency will become very thick; reduce the heat a bit while you keep stirring. As soon as thick airy bubbles appear, or when while scratching the bottom the line stays visible for a few seconds, you'll know the syrup is done! Use the silicon spatula to transfer the syrup into the container. Be careful, it's really hot! More water will evaporate when the liquid cools down, and when the substance reaches room temperature, you will see that it has become a beautiful, thick syrup.

Making the waffle | Weigh 25 grams of fiber and put it into a bowl. Add a pinch of salt, 10 grams buckwheat flour, a pinch of baking powder and 1/2 teaspoon of rapeseed oil. Mix the ingredients together and make a ball. When too dry, add a bit more oil. When too wet, add a bit more buckwheat flour. Bake the waffle on a preheated iron (180 °C) for 1 minute and 15 seconds.

Combine | Take the waffle off the iron and place it on the cutting board. Use a knife to slice it open so that you have two parts. Use a spoon or spatula to add a layer of syrup and cover with the other side of the waffle. Enjoy!

Ingredients
(for 10 waffles)

- 1 kg carrots
- pinch of salt
- 2 tbs rapeseed oil
- 100 g buckwheat flour
- 2 g baking-powder

Material

- juicer
- knife
- cutting board
- 3 bowls
- nut milk bag or clean dish towel
- small sieve
- whisk
- metal spatula
- scale
- large pan
- small container for syrup
- waffle iron

Tip: the bigger the surface of the pan, the faster the water inside the juice can evaporate!

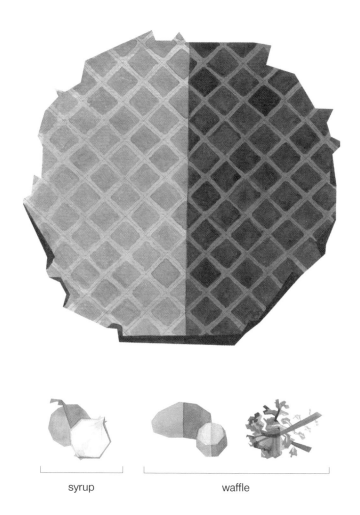

syrup   waffle

Dutch stew stroopwafel

Onion syrup with a potato and kale waffle.

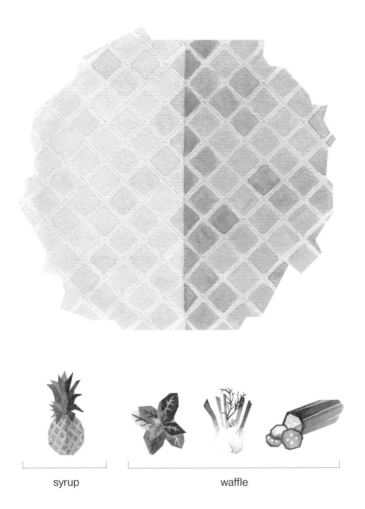

syrup | waffle

Summer stroopwafel

Pineapple syrup with a fresh fennel, cucumber and mint waffle.

4.

Digestive Food

Why undigested food is at the core of food waste.

Food waste is getting a lot of attention lately, and for good reason. You may be surprised to hear that the world produces 17% more food than it did 30 years ago, yet nearly half of that produce never reaches our bellies. Sure, we are using our creativity to think up innovative solutions that can help us reduce, reuse and recycle food waste, but what about over-consumption? Or, on an even smaller scale, the inefficient digestion and nutrient absorption of food by our bodies? Our understanding of "food waste" might be rather narrow-minded.

I believe that instead of worrying about external food waste issues throughout the food chain, we should begin looking more critically at our own eating habits. And in doing so, take a closer look at how the body functions, in order to identify the enormous amounts of food we are wasting—in ways we would never usually regard as waste.

A rather narrow-minded take on food waste

Today, the concept of food waste includes food discarded in factories or in the fields, food not sold in shops or restaurants, and plate waste. However, zooming in on food waste, I was surprised to learn that most people absorb only 75% of the nutrients they consume. For us it's quite "natural" to eat high amounts of processed foods; it's part of our modern diets. Yet our bodies are not designed to process such high quantities of heavy, nutrient-dense foods, and as a result we have difficulty digesting it all at once.

The fact of the matter is that digestion processes of one nutrient group can interfere with and disturb the digestion processes of other nutrient groups. This can lead to unprocessed food in our bellies, causing unbalanced intestinal flora and resulting in inefficient nutrient absorption. This also explains why many people suffer from digestive problems, heartburn and constipation—undigested food is not only a waste of resources; it also damages our health.

A new eating system

Consider the human body as a machine that needs energy to run—this energy comes from our food. Food is our fuel, and as with a car's engine, the more efficiently we process the fuel, the greater the distances we can bridge. The process of gaining energy from this fuel relies on its metabolically active ingredients, which are processed in our digestive system.

We digest nutrients in a specific order, at specific sites, with specific digestive enzymes. In our mouths, the digestion of carbohydrates begins. Then the body processes proteins and lipids, and finally, micro-nutrients (vitamins and minerals).

This led me to wonder why our food isn't designed with this system in mind. If we produced food in the order of its ultimate digestion, our bodies could in theory harvest the full potential of the nutrients' energy, without losing nutritional value in the process of digestion. Perhaps food as it is now just isn't the right fuel for our engines?

Perhaps food as it is now just isn't the right fuel for our engines?

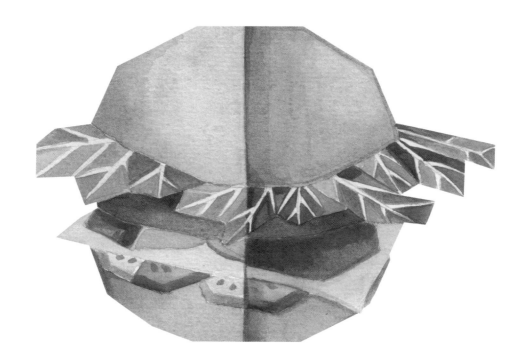

100% nutrients in

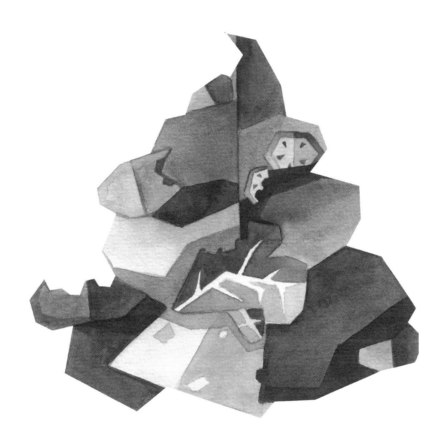

25% nutrients out

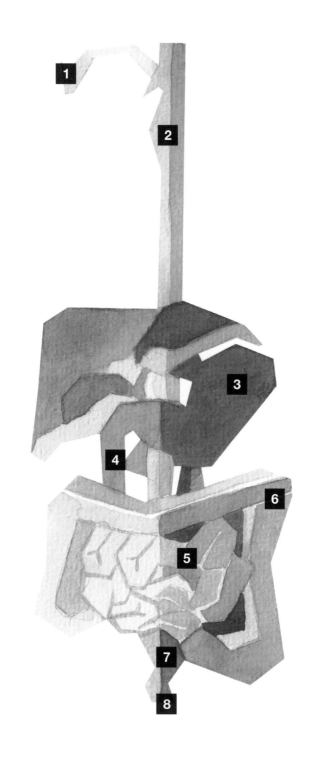

What happens to the food we eat after it enters our body—all the way from mouth to toilet?

The human digestive system

In designing such a new eating system, the logical first step is to investigate how digestion works:

1. Mouth | While chewing the food to make it small enough to swallow, saliva is added. An enzyme in our saliva, amylase, activates the digestion of carbohydrates.

2. Esophagus | This organ transports the chewed food from mouth to stomach.

3. Stomach | The acidity in the stomach deactivates the amylase, which stops the digestion of carbohydrates. The enzyme peptase is released, activating the digestion of proteins.

4. Duodenum | Pancreatic juices inside the duodenum neutralize the acidic mass from the stomach. Peptase is deactivated and the digestion of proteins stops. Bile acids from the gallbladder emulsify the fats before they are digested by the enzyme lipase.

5. Small intestine | The first nutrients are absorbed into the bloodstream. Digestive juices help break down the food into even smaller particles before they move on to the colon.

6. Colon | Absorption of the remaining available nutrients, such as bile salts and electrolytes. Intestinal bacteria dissolves the last food remnants and undigested food. Uptake of vitamin K, B1, B2, B12.

7. Rectum | Here, the feces are collected.

8. Anus | Excretion of feces.

How can we design
a new eating system
to solve food waste
from the inside out,
while improving
both physical
and mental health?

Digestive Food

Looking at how the digestive system works allows us to speculate on how digital fabrication methods—like food printing or encapsulation—could be applied to produce highly efficient "food capsules." Separating the function of eating from the sensory experience. Digestive Food explores the use of encapsulation techniques to balance our intestinal flora, aiming to make food absorption and digestion more efficient.

In these capsules, the nutrients would be layered in order of digestion; similar to functional medicine, nutrient layers are separated by membranes that can only dissolve once the right digestive juices are present to digest the next nutrient layer. This means that in theory, our body would have more time to digest and absorb the food it consumes.

1. Basic capsule

The basic capsule will measure about 5 millimeters in diameter and be built from carbohydrates, protein, lipids and micro-nutrients—in order of digestion. The capsules are small enough that only the carbohydrate layer can be chewed.

2. Carbohydrate wrapper

As the amylase in our saliva activates the digestion of carbohydrates in the mouth anyway, the carbohydrate layer could also be used as a wrapper instead. Filled with capsules of protein, lipids and micro-nutrients, it can change the eating experience and mouth-feel of the food.

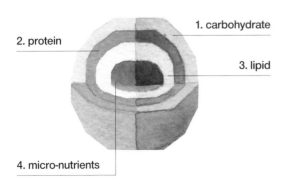

2. protein

1. carbohydrate

3. lipid

4. micro-nutrients

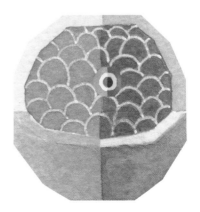

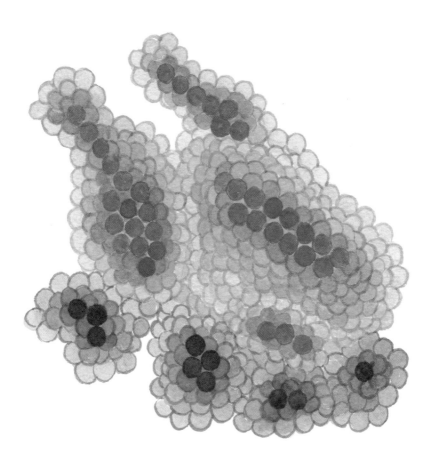

Basic capsule "chicken"

How are we supposed to eat a handful of tiny food capsules of which only the carbohydrate layer can be chewed on? How many will we need to substitute for a normal meal? We could cluster the capsules to either rebuild our existing food, or create entirely new shapes. A new eating system will take some time to get used to but also creates an opportunity to redesign our food!

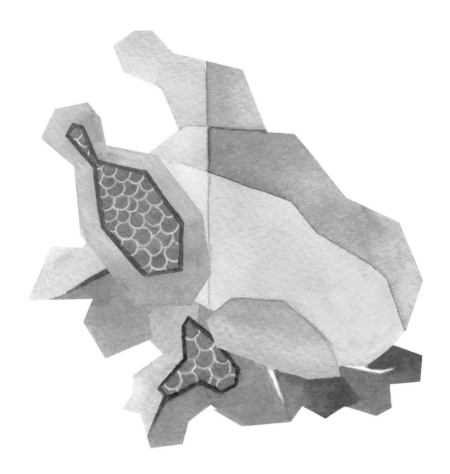

Carbohydrate-wrapped "chicken"

Don't we all love the mouthfeel and sound of chewing on something crunchy? The primitive urge to rip off pieces of food with our teeth? To recreate these pleasures, the carbohydrate layer can be used as a wrapper for the capsules. A membrane around the protein layer will make sure the capsules remain intact until they have reached the stomach.

Personalize your diet

Generally speaking, our current diet consists of approximately 45-60% carbs, 15-20% protein and 20-35% lipids—although not everyone has the same nutritional needs or goals. This technology would allow us to personalize the composition of our diets by simply changing the proportions of the nutrient layers. For example, an athlete in need of a lot of energy could increase the amount of carbohydrates in his diet. If you're looking to gain muscle instead, you can simply reduce the percentage of lipids in your diet and increase the percentage of proteins. In addition, the amount of micro-nutrients—and perhaps even additional medicine—could be manually adjusted before printing your personalized digestive food. Digestive Food could be specifically interesting for certain target groups including astronauts, elderly people and the severely ill.

But however sustainable, functional or healthy the Digestive Food is, if we want people to embrace this new eating system, the food needs to have a certain look, feel, and not least, flavor. How to turn a highly functional eating system consisting mainly of tiny capsules into something delicious?

Why not enrich the eating experience by "seasoning" the food with customized smells, textures, colors and crunch?

Flavor is the sum of taste, smell and texture. Researchers have found that nearly 80% of a food's flavor is determined by its retronasal odor (smelling through your mouth). The smell of food helps us to identify complex flavors and associate them with strongly rooted memories of food. Without smell, we would only be able to identify the five basic tastes: salty, bitter, sweet, sour and umami. In addition to this, the texture, shape, color and sound of food all strongly influence our perception of the flavor.

So, if the look and basic taste of the capsules is not appetizing enough, why not enrich the eating experience by "seasoning" the food with customized smells, textures, colors and crunch, with the help of digital fabrication technologies?

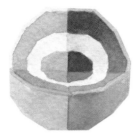

Low carb diet
for losing weight

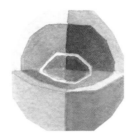

High protein diet
for gaining muscle

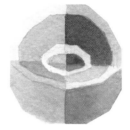

Low fat diet
for losing weight

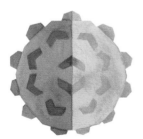

Sweet
rounded, pink, smooth.

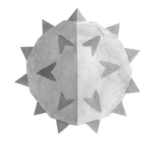

Sour
spiky, yellow/green.

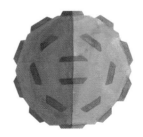

Umami
edged, organge/brown.

Imagine an era in which farmers own nutrient tanks instead of farmland.

Harvesting macro- and micronutrients

As most ingredients in our current food system consist of at least two macro-nutrient groups (fish = protein and fat, mushrooms = proteins and carbs), this makes them unsuitable for the creation of the digestive food capsules. But today, scientists are already making smart use of genetically modified bacteria to create sustainable essences though the natural process of fermentation (think of the creation of citrus extracts through fermentation of modified bacteria instead of large quantities of orange peels).

Why not use this same method for the production of macro- and micronutrients? Imagine an era in which farmers own nutrient tanks instead of farmland. After the nutrients are produced, they will be harvested, dried and stored in cartridges, which afterwards can be used to manufacture the Digestive Food capsules.

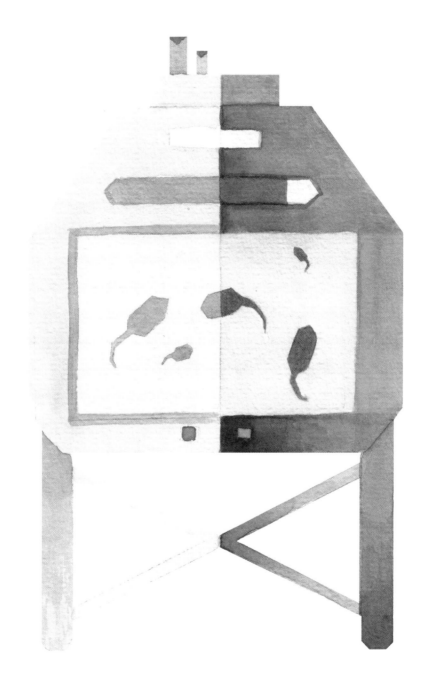

Harvesting carbohydrates instead of carrots

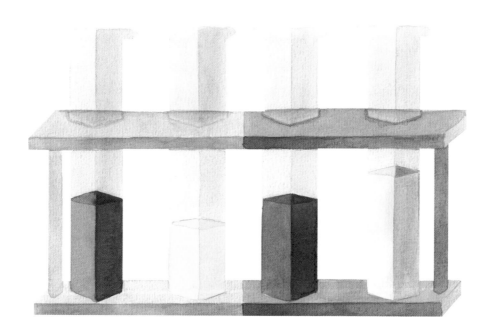

DIY Amylase experiment

To understand the theory behind the Digestive Food project you can try this amylase experiment at home. The experiment visualizes the first steps of the digestion of carbohydrates, starting in the mouth, due to the enzyme amylase in our saliva. In four simple steps, you will gain an understanding of how starch is turned into glucose.

Instructions

1. Fill each test tube with a thumb length of potato liquid (contains starch), and number the tubes 1 to 4.

2. Use a clean pipette to add three drops of iodine to tube 1. Use the other pipette to add three drops of Fehling's reagent to tube 3. Shake the tubes. What happens to the liquid and why?

3. Empty the contents of tubes 2 and 4 in your mouth and gargle the potato fluid for at least one minute. Spit the liquid back into the test tubes (you can use the funnel for this).

4. Add three drops of iodine to tube 2, and three drops of Fehling's reagent to tube 4. Make sure you use the right pipette. Shake the tubes. What happens to the starch water and why?

Explanation

Tube 1 | will turn dark brown because the iodine reacts to the presence of starch in the potato liquid.

Tube 2 | will turn orange/brown, the natural color of iodine mixed with water. This displays the absence of starch due to the amylase in our saliva, which turned the starch into glucose.

Tube 3 | will turn bright blue, the natural color of diluted Fehling's reagent when dissolved in water.

Tube 4 | will turn light purple, displaying the presence of glucose as a result of the first step of the digestion of carbohydrates in the mouth from starch to glucose.

What you need

- 4 test tubes
- test tube rack
- 2 small pipettes
- marker
- small funnel
- potato liquid*
- Iodine
- Fehling's reagent

*boil one small potato in 150ml water, then sieve the cooking liquid and pour it into a bottle.

Indicators

Iodine | reacts to starch by turning a solution black.

Fehlings reagent | reacts to glucose by turning a solution light purple.

Beyond Taboos

5.

The Other Dinner

How eating mice could stimulate innovation

Back in the days before animals were treated as meat factories, meat was a delicacy exclusively available to the rich. The entire animal was eaten, from nose to tail; no part was wasted. Knowledge of how to prepare each part was passed down from generation to generation. However, with the rise of modernity (and with it, industrialization), we could suddenly afford to eat only the "good parts" of the animal, and much of this knowledge was lost. And as a result, we became spoiled and picky when it came to ourw meat.

As the global population grows and the demand for meat increases, we will need to broaden our perspective if we want to continue eating meat. Even though the "meatless meats" on the market today are more flavorful and varied than in years past, plant- or insect-based meats are not "real" meat. In vitro meat (meat grown in a lab from the stem cells of an animal) could be a viable alternative to meet the market's demand. In 2013, the first in vitro meat hamburger made from cow cells was presented to the public, and today many food startups in Silicon Valley and Israel are actively exploring the potential of this technology (think lab-grown duck chorizo and foie gras). But while most of our current meat comes from highly domesticated and carefully bred species, many people still fear eating "lab-engineered" meat. Let's stop applying double standards; it's about time we get rid of our prejudices and cultural taboos.

How cultural taboos hinder scientific innovation

Much of meat's taste comes from the combination of its muscle tissue (influenced by the animal's movement in life) with blood vessels and fat content. Today, in vitro meat consists solely of muscle tissue, which means it has little taste, texture and color (this is added).
If our goal is to grow pure protein from muscle weave, wouldn't it be more logical to use the most efficient cells to do so? Stem cells of mice, for example, grow much faster and more efficiently into muscle tissue than cows' cells. So why do scientists not use mice cells instead, in theory saving time, energy and costs?

"In theory 10 embryonic stem cells could multiply up to 50.000.000 cells within two months. Because embryonic cells have an unlimited capacity to renew themselves, one production line could - in theory - feed the entire world. At this point certain production lines are only developed from mouse, monkey, rat and human cells while embryonic stem cells from livestock have the tendency to change into specialized neuron cells."

- Bernard Roelen cellbiologist, Utrecht University

Much of our attitude towards meat is culturally determined and rests on cultural taboos: In the Netherlands and in many other Western countries, eating mice is simply not done. The same goes for eating pigs' legs, brains and cockles. In that context, in vitro meat is already a big leap for the ordinary citizen to make, let alone in vitro meat grown from mice. Such an idea would struggle to find acceptance in our society.

If we only decided to break down these taboos and open our mouths to "other" (parts of) animals, and generally redefine what we regard as "meat," researchers in food science departments would be able to base their experiments on efficiency and costs, rather than the consumer's picky appetite.

Can we stimulate innovation by removing cultural taboos?

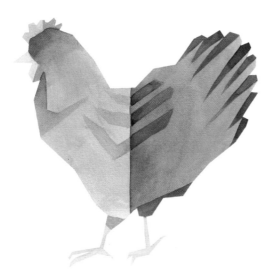

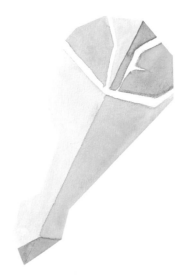

2013 | Until recently, the only option to eat a piece of meat was to slaughter the entire animal. Now, lab-grown hamburgers, duck chorizo and foie gras are a fact.

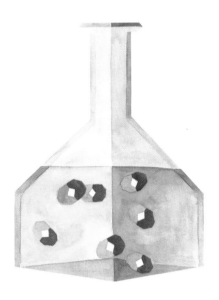

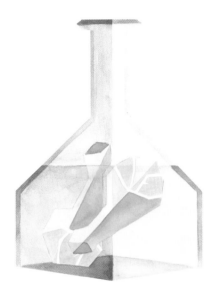

2020 How long before we can grow an entire chicken wing including skin and bones?

How to cook the entire animal

I must admit that I too had a rather limited view on eating meat. I mean, didn't we all grow up with pre-packaged square pieces of meat from the supermarket? Time to change that, and start a culinary adventure into the past, present and future of meat. The book Odd Bits: How to Cook the Rest of the Animal, by Jennifer McLagan, guided me in the beginning of my research. I wanted to understand why we no longer eat the weird parts, why eating mice is taboo, and how cultured meat is actually made. After all, how can we form an opinion on whether lab-grown meat is a good alternative for the future if we have no idea how it is made and how it tastes?

The Other Dinner - The project

To give myself and other people an opportunity for hands-on exploration I organized an experimental event; The Other Dinner. A public event to discuss the future of meat and the impact cultural taboos have on innovation. Divided into three chapters, we questioned the past, present and future of meat. Each chapter challenged the participants to become more tolerant towards alternative protein consumption and helped them to form an opinion based not only on facts, but on personal experience.

In preparation for the first part, I gathered six recipes designed to quickly expand the limited range of meats we are used to eating. As it was rather ambitious to kick off with decanting and filling a pig's leg, frying pork cracklings and bone marrow seemed like a good start.

The six recipes

1 | Pork cracklings
Fried slices of pig skin seasoned with rosemary.

2 | Bone marrow
Crispy bread pockets filled with hot creamy bone marrow.

3 | Cibreo
Stew from offal with white wine sauce.

4 | Cervello fritto
Fried calf brains.

5 | Zampone di Modena
Pig trotter filled with the skin, ears and tail of the pig served with lentils and mashed potatoes.

6 | Pig head
Roasted pig head with carrot stew.

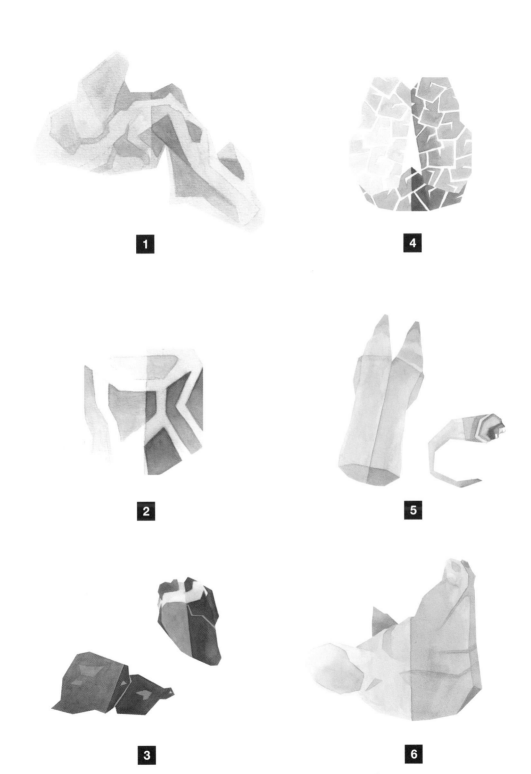

1

4

2

5

3

6

Part 1 - The other parts

"The other parts" was an exploration of cooking the often-undesired parts of the animal, aiming to expand the range of meats we eat today. The plan was to make two dishes every week over the course of one month, starting off with the most accessible recipes, the ingredients of which were easy to obtain. Note that in the Netherlands, pig ears and tails are directly sent to China—where people eat them as a delicacy. Imagine the hassle I had to go through getting that pig's head... Because the animal parts had to be ordered from different butchers, it took quite some time to arrange the full list of ingredients.

In many countries the head is considered the best part of an animal; it contains a wealth of different flavors and textures. Eating an animal head is regarded a symbol of power—a man's mastery over a beast during the hunting season. Yet in the Netherlands, pig heads are only used for making brawn and broth. Due to legislation, adult pigs' heads are never sold in one piece.

I realized during the cooking process that I was constantly moving further out of my comfort zone; flushing off blood and removing hair and ear wax from a pig's head were not yet part of my skill set at that point.

Never before had I cleaned the ears of my food.

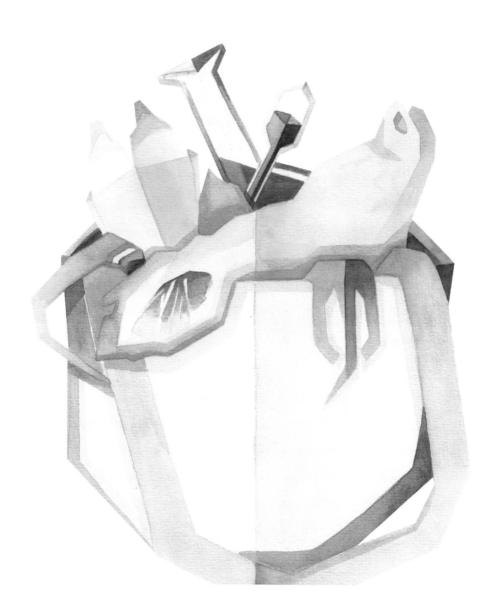

The 'other parts' of the animal

An anatomy lesson

Armed with a bag of legs, ears and tails, an anatomy lesson awaited me. In order to make traditional Zampone di Modena, I needed a deboned pig trotter. Obviously I couldn't get my hands on that item, as we don't eat the dish in the Netherlands. I had to figure out how to get the bones and flesh out of the leg while keeping the skin intact. I can tell you, this was quite the challenge—but as they say, practice makes perfect. So here are some tips to get you started.

How to debone a pig trotter

1. Place the trotter in salt water for a few hours. The skin will become softer and cleaner. Use a scalpel to make an incision on the back of the trotter so that it will be easier to turn the skin inside out.

2. Start at the top of the trotter by pulling on the skin and cutting the meat/fat as close to the skin as possible. Eventually, you can pull the skin down and turn it as a sock around the bottom part. The skin stretches more this way, so it will be easier to cut loose.

3. Once you reached the toes, the most difficult part begins. You need to know where to cut and how the bones and cartilage are connected to the skin. Carefully try to cut around the bones—you want the skin to remain intact. (The smallest toe can't be removed, you will leave this part in the Zampone.) When the skin is loose, turn it back to normal and use kitchen wire to stitch the sides back together so you get a nice sleeve to fill.

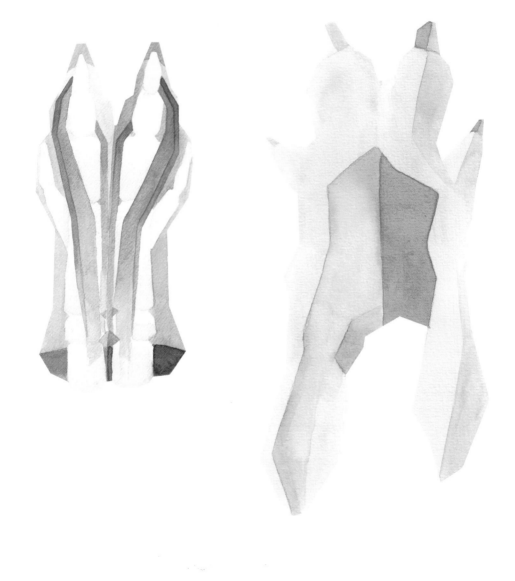

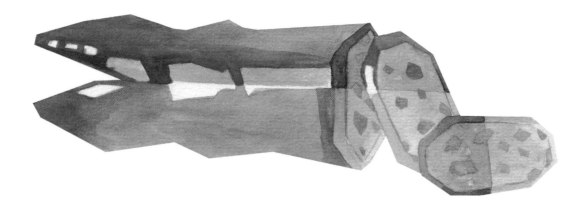

Zampone di Modena

Pig trotter filled with the skin, ears and tail of the pig

Zampone was invented in the sixteenth century (1511), when the troops of Pope Julius
II besieged Mirandola. The citizens were afraid the troops would take their pigs, so they
slaughtered them and stuffed the meat inside the skin and legs. Before stuffing, they minced
and seasoned the meat to preserve it. After winter, the sausages were boiled, sliced into pieces
and eaten. This way Zampone (stuffed leg) and Cotechino (stuffed skin) were created. In the
next century, these dishes became a specialty, and the recipe has been improved on and
adjusted ever since. Zampone and Cotechino make proper use of many parts of the pig and
have become traditional Christmas and New Year's Eve dishes. The sausages are traditionally
eaten with mashed potatoes or lentils.

Instructions

1. Use a torch to remove the remains of hair on the meat. Rinse the tail, skin, leg and shoulder meat with cold water and pat them dry with a paper towel. If not already done, stitch the skin of the leg together with needle and thread, leaving one small opening for the stuffing. Place the leg in the refrigerator. Cut the skin and the shoulder meat into pieces. Try to cut the skin and meat off the tail.

2. Grind the fat meat (skin and tail) with a wide grinding plate and use a smaller grinding plate to mince the shoulder meat to create a nice texture. Place the minced meat in a steel bowl.

3. When all the meat is minced, add the spices and mix everything together. Take the leg out of the refrigerator and stuff it with the minced meat.

4. Knit the ends of the leg together with a needle and kitchen wire. When closed, wrap the linen cloth around the leg and spiral some kitchen wire around the cloth to tighten it.

5. Place the leg in hot water with 3 tsp salt and let it cook for 2 hours. A brown oily layer will appear on the water. After 2 hours, you can take the Zampone out of the pot and slice it into pieces of 1cm. Serve the Zampone with lentils or mashed potatoes.

Ingredients

- 200 g pork shoulder
- 200 g pork skin
- 1 pork leg without bone
- 2 pork tails
- 2 tsp cinnamon
- 2 tsp pimenta
- 2 tsp black pepper
- 1 pinch nutmeg
- 30 g sea salt

Materials needed

- meat mincer
- spoon
- cutting plate
- knife
- large cooking pot
- kitchen wire
- needle
- unstained linen cloth
- kitchen torch
- cooking plate

Part 2 - The other animal

After the intense experience of cooking with the "other" parts, I took on the second challenge, "The other animal," and thus started to experiment with eating mice. As it was my goal to normalize eating in vitro mouse meat, it seemed like a good first step to try regular mouse meat first. To make the idea more palatable, I created mouse liver parfait bonbons. This was a subtle way of combining the unwanted with the desired. Obviously, there were no recipes online for mouse liver parfait bonbons, and so I looked for liver-parfait recipes and simply adjusted them.

Eating rats and mice is a big taboo in most cultures due to fear of disease or religious prohibition. However, in some cultures rats and mice form a dietary staple and an important source of animal protein. According to old myths, eating rat meat can prevent and cure back pains. In Africa, mice are captured in cornfields and dried, pickled or grilled before being sold as street food.

Now, where to buy the mouse livers? Well, the short answer is nowhere, because mice are not on our menu. Eventually, I found a kilogram of frozen mice in a reptile shop, which I defrosted in order to extract the livers. In doing so, instead of finding one liver inside one mouse, I found four! It turns out mice have four livers.

I baked and mixed the livers with herbs and double cream into a parfait, and used it together with a bit of cranberry compote as filling for a dark chocolate bonbon. They tasted both savory and sweet. A pretty good first encounter with eating mice, if you ask me.

Did you know that mice have four livers?

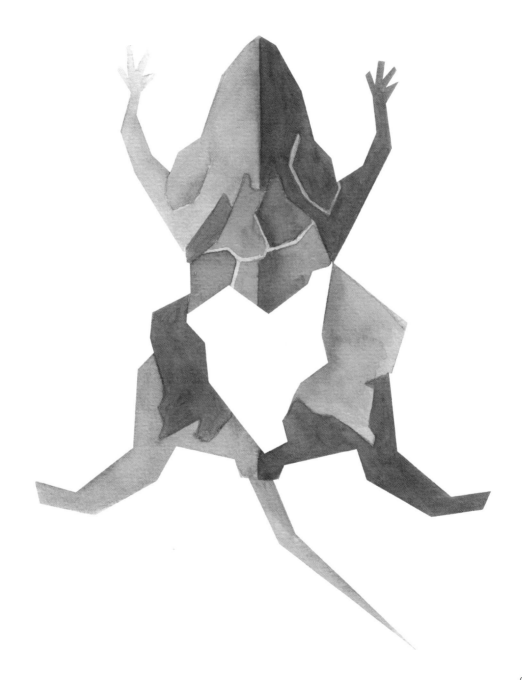

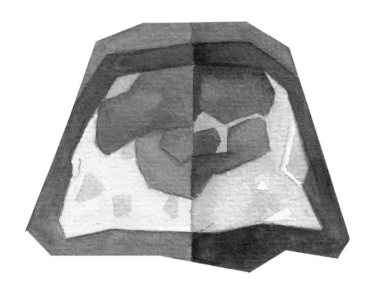

Recipe | Mouse liver parfait bonbons

The slightly sweet, but bitter taste of the cranberries complete the dark chocolate
and nutty wild taste of the mice-liver parfait very well. You can use this recipe
as a guideline to mix and match the liver parfait with anything you like.

Instructions

Note: Place the mice two hours before preparation into a bowl with cold water and salt to soak the skin and clean them.

Preparation | Take the mice out of the bowl, dry them with paper towels and place them on the cutting board. Put on a pair of gloves and skin the mouse, starting with an incision from neck to tail. Separate the muscle meat and livers from the rest of the mouse and place them into a bowl.

To make the parfait | Chop a shallot and fry the pieces in a pan with butter, over medium heat. Add the mouse meat and livers, some thyme, and cook everything until the livers are brown but still pink on the inside. Place the meat in a food processor and mix briefly. Boil the Madeira in the pan which was used to cook the meat and pour it into the food processor. Add the cream, butter, salt and ginger as well, and mix until smooth. Pour the mixture into a bowl and place it into the refrigerator until it has set.

To make the bonbon | Melt half the chocolate au-bain-marie and fill the mold with a small layer of chocolate. It's important that all sides of the mold are covered with chocolate as well. Place the mold briefly into the refrigerator until the chocolate is solid.

Take a small spoon and add a thin layer of cranberry compote. Take the parfait out of the refrigerator and add a layer of parfait. Melt the remaining chocolate to fill up the mold. Place the mold back into the refrigerator and wait for the chocolate to become solid.

Your mouse liver parfait bonbon is finished and can be eaten. The bonbon is delicious with coffee, but we advise a nice glass of scotch or port!

Ingredients

(+/-15 chocolates)

- livers and meat of four mice
- 75 g butter
- 1 small shallot
- 1 tsp thyme
- 50 mL Madeira
- 75 mL double cream
- ½ tsp salt
- ¼ tsp ground ginger
- 200 g dark chocolate dark
- cranberry compote

Material

- frying pan
- knife
- cutting board
- whisk
- spoon
- very sharp scalpel
- au bain marie pan
- gloves
- spatula
- food processor
- chocolate mold
  for 15 chocolates

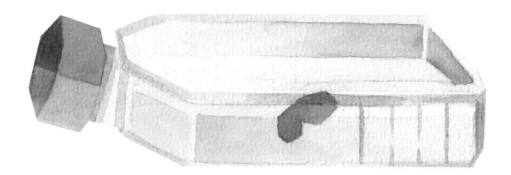

Part three - In vitro meat

On to the final stage: In vitro meat. Together with a DIY biotechnologist we experimented with the tissue cultures of various mice cells. Then we wrote a recipe, based on the actual protocol of scientists, on how to make your own in vitro mouse meat, to give consumers a better idea of how this meat is made. In addition, it gives them the opportunity to start experimenting with tissue culturing themselves.

While we never ate the tissue cultures, we did succeed in getting some liver and muscle cells to multiply. We closely monitored the cell cultures with a microscope to see how they were doing. Following the protocol and trying to make in vitro meat ourselves was a weighty experience. It helped me understand the technology and allowed me to form a constructive opinion on in vitro meat as potential future food.

Experiment | DIY In vitro mice meat

Instructions

Proper hygiene and sterile conditions are crucial to successful cell culturing. Wash your hands and sterilize your equipment by boiling it in a pressure cooker for at least 25 minutes. Use 70% ethanol to clean a workbench and move slowly to reduce the airflow that might carry bacteria and fungi. Perform all procedures below as close to a flame as possible.

1. Prepare the Ham's F12 medium by supplementing it with 5% penicillin & streptomycin antibiotics and 5% serum (preferably bovine calf serum).

2. Allocate 10 mL of medium each in three red-capped 20 mL culture flasks. Label the flasks with the letters E, S and K respectively.

3. Put on a pair of (nitrile) gloves and put the mouse in a petri dish. Using a sterile scalpel, start an incision from neck to tail. Three types of tissue need to be obtained: 1) epithelial cells, which can be found in between organs and underneath the skin; 2) skeletal muscle cells; 3) kidney cells. Cut a small piece of tissue and transfer it into the culture flask with sterile tweezers.

4. Incubate the tissue culture at 37° C in a 5% CO_2 incubator for at least 24 hours.

5. After 24 hours you can place a little bit of fluid from the tissue culture flask onto a microscope slide and cover it. Make sure you use a sterile pipette tip and hold a blue flame next to the flask when opening it. If you do this every few days and compare it under the microscope, you can see if the cells are actually growing inside of the medium.

Ingredients

- 1 mouse
- ethanol 70%
- Ham's F12
- penicillin
- streptomycin
- distillate water
- bovine calf serum

Materials needed

- petri dish
- 3 coated 20 mL culture flasks
- very sharp scalpel
- nitrile gloves
- tweezers
- pipette
- pipette tips
- pressure cooker
- paper towels
- disinfectant
- ethanol siphon
- torch
- lighter
- incubator
- marker

The Other Dinner - The result

The aim of The Other Dinner was to provide an opportunity for a very diverse group of people to experience nose to tail cooking, eating other animals and creating their own cultured meat.

Participants found that after doing hands-on work themselves they were much more willing to taste the experimental meat dishes. The fact that the dinner was a social activity fueled by peer pressure also helped a lot. "After having worked with the strange animal parts for some hours, it almost becomes normal." one of the participants responded. This was exactly the reaction I was hoping for.

The morning and afternoon program (parts 1 & 2) opened up their minds to considering a future including in vitro meat—and since they had already eaten mice and muskrats anyway, they couldn't care less whether scientists would use cells from mice or cows for the creation of cultured meat in the future.

"After having worked with the strange animal parts for some hours, it almost becomes normal."

- participant The Other Dinner

Beyond chops and steaks

Consider how in the future, we may no longer have to raise an entire animal to eat its meat; we could simply grow the parts we like from harvested cells inside a petri dish. This way, we will be able to pet the living animal, while eating it!

Just imagine the possibilities. We're not just talking regular chops and steaks here. Perhaps you've always dreamt of a kidney steak or juicy epithelium patch? Or what about using preserved DNA from extinct animals to create dodo meat or dinosaur nuggets? This technology may hold the potential to reshape our long-lasting relationship with meat, and that's probably a good thing.

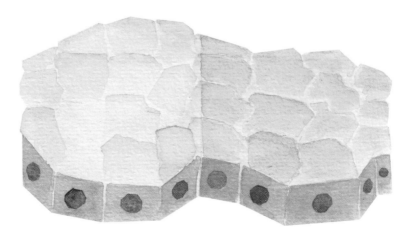

Our current meat is not sustainable due to its inefficient protein conversion rate, the production of greenhouse gases, and the need for massive areas of agricultural land. If the world wants to continue eating meat, we are going to need alternatives. Scientists believe that in vitro meat might prove a good replacement for current meat products. They predict that "cultured meat" will eventually use far less water and energy and can reduce CO_2 emissions by 96%.

In vitro meat is meat grown outside the body of a living organism. The basic principle is that one stem cell multiplies into many stem cells, after which these cells specialize into muscle cells and form large muscle fibers which eventually become meat. But in a world in which meat is scarce, how far will consumers be willing to go to continue eating meat?

6.

In vitro ME

How far are you willing to go
to continue eating meat?

Our ancestors were hunter-gatherers, and among their distinguishing characteristics was the habit of actively killing animals for meat. Food was their first priority and took up most of their time and energy. This is not something we have to worry about today; we simply buy our meat from a butcher or at the supermarket. Yet as the world population increases and the demand for meat continues to grow, this passive attitude must change.

A different mindset

Today, we take for granted the separation of producer and consumer: If you're not part of the production or growth of the food, all you have to do is buy and eat it. Through industrialization, mass production and legislation our food has become safe, relatively inexpensive and available on practically every corner. We no longer eat because we are hungry; we eat just because we like it.

How far are you willing to go to continue eating meat?

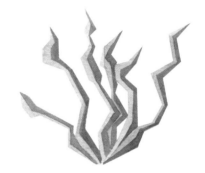

Luckily, an ever-growing part of the world population is becoming more aware of how personal food choices affect their health, the environment and animal welfare. People realize that it's time for a change. To stop eating animal products, start buying locally grown produce, or even start their own vegetable garden in order to get closer to the food they are consuming. This also relates to the production of alternative proteins and meat substitutes, such as those made from beans, algae, insects or cultured meat. Yet the majority of people still eat meat. How to address that?

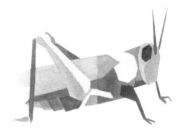

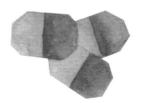

Taking responsibility

At present, in vitro meat is the only meat alternative not made from plants or insects but instead regarded as "real" meat. But it's expensive, takes a long time to grow, and more importantly, it needs to pass legislation before it can go on the market. Until that day arrives, I wonder how far people are willing to go themselves to continue eating meat. Would it influence the consumer's decision if they played an active role in the production of meat—that is, if they realized how much energy and raw material it takes to produce a piece of meat? Would a meat eater be willing to use their own body as a production site? Would they be willing to grow meat from their own muscle tissue?

In Vitro ME - The concept

In Vitro ME is a personal bioreactor-jewel which enables the production of human muscle tissue—a speculative design project to make people aware of the resources needed to produce meat. Since it will most likely cost us more energy to produce human meat than we will gain from consuming it, the process cannot be considered very efficient. But the question is, should it be efficient?

The personal bioreactor-jewel nestles down on your chest, where it cultivates human muscle tissue. The direct connection between the body and the bioreactor enables the exchange of heat, nutrients, oxygen and waste substances in order to create "personal meat" for consumption. In other words, the jewel uses your body as a production site. Fed with your own blood and "trained" according to your level of activity, this self-grown meat is a direct translation of your lifestyle. This way, you literally eat what you are and are what you eat.

**Would you be willing
to use your own body
as a production site
to grow meat from your
own muscle tissue?**

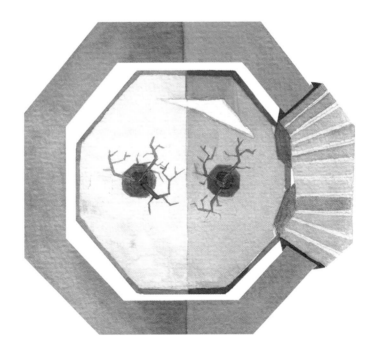

How it works

Myoblasts (a cluster of muscle cells) obtained from human muscle tissue are placed onto the amulet, laying on top of a 3D-printed edible grid (myoblasts are preferable to stem cells, as they are certain to grow into muscle cells). The printed grid contains an artificial vascular system, which is connected to one's own vascular system; this allows for blood to flow and substances to diffuse in and out of the myoblast cells. As oxygen and nutrients are obtained through our vascular system, the waste substances (such as CO_2) are released back into the blood circulation and filtered inside our body. Throughout this process, the cells receive the same amount of substance as they would receive in vivo (inside the body).

You are what you eat

Traditional in vitro meat is "trained" with electrical pulses. Yet, as the bioreactor is attached to the human body, the amulet's effigies are trained similarly to how animal muscle tissue is trained through physical exercise. Scientists are also working on new methods for muscle training; they have learned that muscle cells (when attached to fixed points inside the grid) can work as Velcro, and as a result, start generating pulses themselves.

Because the myoblasts inside the bioreactor are fed and trained by the human body, the product directly reflects the wearer's current physical state. Perhaps this will stimulate people to take better care of their bodies, health and diet—and in doing so, gradually increasing the quality of the meat.

Because the myoblasts inside the bioreactor are fed and trained by the human body, the product directly reflects the wearer's current physical state.

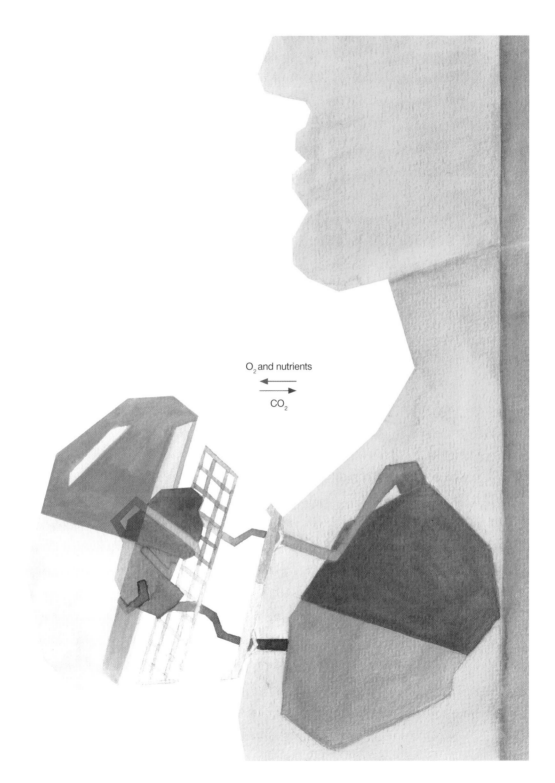

O_2 and nutrients

CO_2

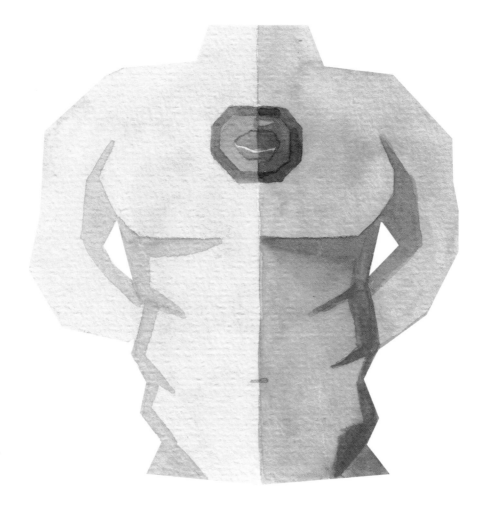

You are what you eat and eat what you are

MIKE'S STEAK

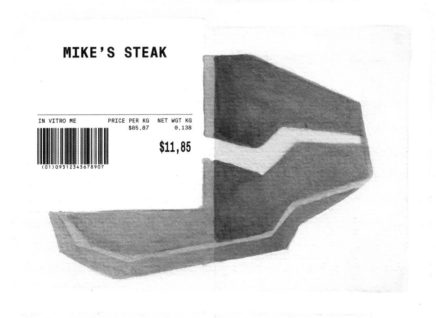

IN VITRO ME	PRICE PER KG	NET WGT KG
	$85,87	0,138

$11,85

(01)09312345678907

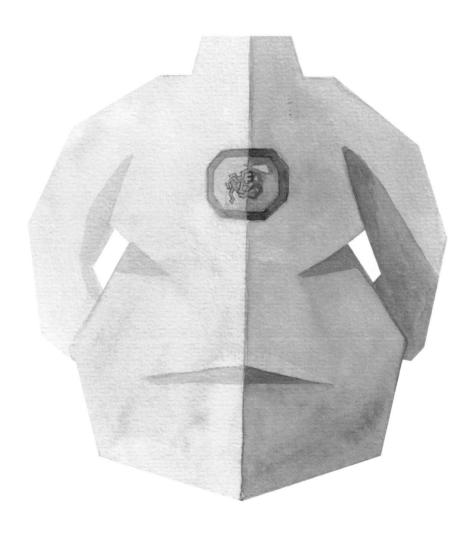

You are what you eat and eat what you are

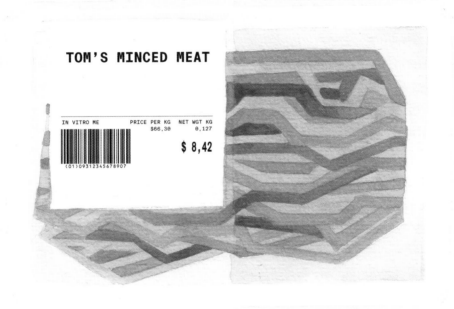

TOM'S MINCED MEAT

IN VITRO ME	PRICE PER KG	NET WGT KG
	$66,30	0,127

$ 8,42

(01)09312345678907

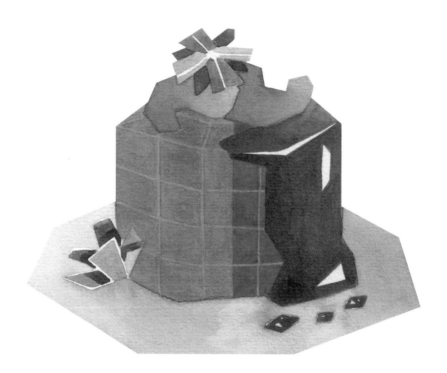

Recipe | In Vitro ME
From the In Vitro Meat Cookbook by Next Nature Network

In this recipe, the porky flavor of human flesh is complemented with a blood-red glaze that lends sensuous notes of earth, sugar and smoke. A more modern, gentler update on centuries-old cannibal rituals, In Vitro ME is best shared with a lover as the ultimate expression of unity.

Instructions

1. Preheat the oven to 180 °C. Mix the maple syrup, broth and beet in a saucepan and bring to a boil. Lower heat and simmer until the glaze has been reduced by half.

2. Melt the butter in a heavy skillet. Add the meat and cook until browned—one to two minutes per side. Transfer the meat to a small baking dish. Pour the glaze over the meat, turning to coat. Bake for 8 to 10 minutes, until an instant-read thermometer inserted in the center reads 57 °C.

3. Remove the meat from the baking dish, put on two serving plates and cover with aluminum foil. Return the glaze to the saucepan and simmer until it is thick and syrupy. Using an immersion blender, blend the glaze until no beet chunks remain.

4. Drizzle the glaze over the In Vitro ME and garnish with the blossoms. Enjoy!

Ingredients

- 2 In Vitro ME effigies
- 60 g butter
- A pinch of salt, pepper and chipotle powder
- 90 mL maple syrup
- 90 mL broth
- 1 small beet, peeled and diced
- 30 mL Worcestershire sauce
- Begonia blossoms

Material

- baking paper
- blender
- big bowl
- ovendish
- saucepan
- scale
- spoon
- whisk

Cannibalism

Would the production and consumption of human in vitro meat constitute cannibalism? "Cannibalism" describes the act of humans eating the flesh or internal organs of other human beings—so does this term apply to eating one's own flesh? Acceptance and personal boundaries will play a major role in the discussion of whether eating self-produced flesh from muscle cells is cannibalism or not.

However, eating human flesh may come with several health risks. Kuru is an example of a fatal brain disease caused by cannibalism, which appeared in the Eastern Highlands province of Papua New Guinea in the 1950s. This means that, even if In Vitro ME were feasible today, it would not be wise to recommend the consumption of human cultured meat at our current stage of evolution.

But who knows where evolution will lead us...

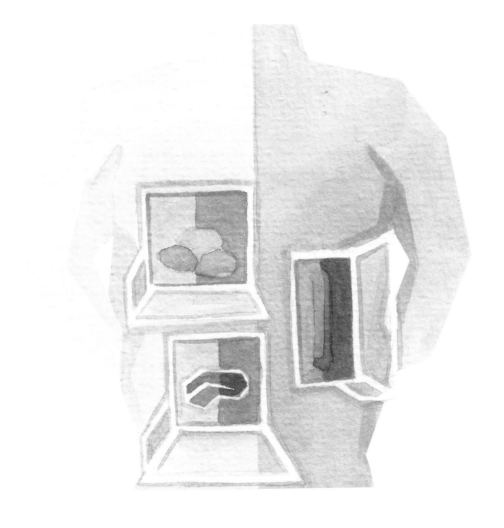

Human 'snackwall' | Grow your own steak, sausage or nugget

Index

5 The Other Dinner (pg 80 - 99)

2013 | Eindhoven University of Technology

Design coach: Janine Huizenga, Next Nature Lab

In collaboration with:

Waag society Amsterdam

Coach | Lucas Evers

DIY biotechnologist | Pieter van Bohemen

First taster | Cecilia Raspanti

Production assistant | Maike Bisseling

Further reading: Odd Bits by Jennifer Mc Lagan

6 In vitro ME (pg 100 - 113)

2013 | Eindhoven University of Technology

Design coach: Menno Stoffelsen, Next Nature Lab

In collaboration with:

Next Nature Network | In Vitro Meat Cookbook, 2014

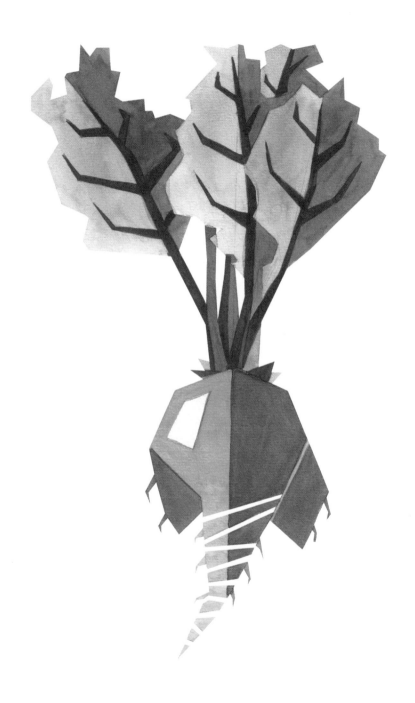

Special thanks to

My fantastic team; Lisa den Teuling, Ruben Baart, Jack Caulfield and Jon Arts | BIS Publishers for being enthusiastic and supportive about the book from day one | My parents and friends who received a million screenshots to comment on | Rebecca Chesney for writing an amazing foreword and Triodos Foundation for their financial support.